Help!
I'm sweating!

All information contained in this book was gathered and carefully checked by the author to the best of his knowledge and ability. Nevertheless, errors in the content cannot be totally excluded. The author and his collaborators assume no responsibility or liability for inaccuracies in the text.

The statements of this adviser that were researched with the greatest care possible and with competent support do not nullify the obligation of critically examining the assertions made in the text, since medical developments are subject to constant progress and change. Obtaining the independent opinion of a medical practitioner of the suitability and risk of a certain form of therapy, of the indications, dosages and possible side effects of a healing procedure is the *conditio sine qua non* in the therapeutic process and necessitates personal discussions with a trained therapist.

Impressum

1st English Edition March 2006

Cover design
bindergrafik – Peter Binder – Erlinsbacherstrasse 94, CH-5000 Aarau, Switzerland
Tel. +41 (0) 62 822 44 11 – Fax +41 (0) 62 822 44 91
E-Mail: info@bildbearbeitung.ch, Internet: www.bildbearbeitung.ch

Author
Dietmar Stattkus in collaboration with Hidrex GmbH
e-mail: dstattkus@transpiration.de – Internet: **www.transpiration.de**
e-mail: info@hidrex.de – Internet: **www.hidrex.de**
translated by **roth@juro-translation.com**

List of image sources
Figures 1-3; © Cognis Deutschland GmbH & Co. KG, Skin Care Forum, edition 25, 36 (www.scf-online.com.)
Figures 4-5: © 2004, Klinik für Dermatologie, Venerologie und Allergologie, Charité-Universitätsmedizin Berlin (http://www.charite.de/ch/derm/info/hy_hi_ einleitung.html)
Figures 7, 8: © Hidrex GmbH
Figures 10, 11: © Prof. Dr. Dr. Dirk Nolte, Praxisklinik für Mund-, Kiefer- und Gesichtschirurgie, Sauerbruchstr. 48, D-81377 München
Figures 6, 9, 12, 13: © PD Dr. med. Christoph Schick, Prinz-Ludwig-Str. 6, D-80333 München (http://www.dhhz.de)

© Dietmar Stattkus 2006
ISBN 3-8334-4150-X
CIP – Title inclusion in the Deutschen Bibliothek [German Library]

Dietmar Stattkus

Help! I'm sweating!

Causes, Phenomena, Therapies

An advisory manual for pathological perspiration

Contents

Advice to the reader

Pathologically increased perspiration, hyperhidrosis, is frequently concealed by its victims and not recognized by physicians. As a result the patient is caught up in a vicious circle causing an almost endless path of suffering.

At the same time numerous possibilities for treatment are available. They range from changing the lifestyle and overcoming stress through topical applications and physical treatments to surgical measures and the ingestion of drugs. The most common manifestation form of excessive perspiration of the hands, feet, and armpits can be treated by following a stepwise plan.

There is international consensus that, in the case of excessive axillary perspiration, first aluminum chloride solutions can be applied externally; if this does not meet with sufficient success, botulinum toxin A can be injected; and finally, if these two forms of therapy fail, the axillary sweat glands can be surgically removed. Suction curettage is especially suited as a gentle yet effective operation.

Tap water iontophoresis is the treatment of choice for excessive perspiration of the hands and feet. A possible alternative for the palms is injection of botulinum toxin A. In extreme cases an improvement can be achieved by taking medications, and as a last resort one may perform a surgical sympathectomy, although this involves certain side effects.

"Help! I'm sweating!" provides the people affected with the opportunity to get to know their affliction, to accept it and to communicate with their surroundings in order to experience healing or at least some relief in cooperation with expert and responsible doctors.

Oldenburg, October 2005

Prof. Dr. Erhard Hölzle
Clinic for Dermatology and Allergology
Oldenburg Clinic, Germany

Hyperhidrosis is not merely a cosmetic problem for those suffering from it but rather it also involves serious occupational, health-related and psychosocial burdens. The present book gives a detailed survey of the causes, forms of clinical manifestation and possible therapies for hyperhidrosis and with its clear and precise mode of presentation contributes to better understanding of the clinical picture.

This clearly understandable compendium is written in a highly stimulating didactic form so that it deserves a broad readership and numerous editions.

Düsseldorf, January 2006

Prof. Dr. Dr. h. c. Thomas Ruzicka
Priv.-Doz. Dr. Daniela Bruch-Gerharz
University Skin Clinic, Düsseldorf, Germany

Preface

The previous editions of the Book *Help! I'm Sweating!* enjoyed a highly favorable response. This is impressively demonstrated by the many letters from readers and the feedback to the home page accompanying the book.

Since the 2nd edition came out a few new facts have emerged relative to clarification and therapy. In addition, an extremely high demand for information still exists so that it appeared necessary to subject the existing version to a thorough revision. New scientific discoveries based on clinical studies and research as well as expanded therapeutic possibilities were incorporated, such as the unpleasant odor of perspiration or body odor which accompanies hyperhidrosis, which further increases the suffering of those afflicted.

Simultaneously with the revision of the book, the desire for translation and international publication of the compendium was complied with. The possibility of including colored illustrations in the digital printing of the book was accepted as a pleasant side effect for the new version so that the subject matter is now presented in a much more visually acceptable form.

Thanks to the popularity and rapid growth of the Internet the disease of excessive perspiration is becoming increasingly less a taboo subject. The freedoms of this medium have fundamentally revolutionized the public health system. In parallel with this progress, necessarily also the pathological phenomenon of excessive perspiration has been made accessible to a broad public.

Thus in the meanwhile there is a large number of serious data sources on the web which permit a better understanding of this recognized disease that must be taken seriously.

Victims can interact in discussion forums, and information previously reserved to medical practitioners can now be called up by everyone. To those interested a medical data bank of tremendous size is now available, which can be expanded and updated in seconds.

And the typology of the victims itself is changing due to the information possibilities of the internet. The once "ignorant" hyperhidrotic who in the past was not infrequently notified by doctors treating him of the lack of effective therapies is now increasingly being transformed into a self-aware and therapeutically cooperating patient, and it is precisely this evolution which the present advisory compendium is intended to promote.

Quality and quantity of clinical therapy have also favorably evolved. Thus, in the meanwhile in many countries, contact sites and institutions exist with competent therapists sensitized to the problem. The result of this steadily increasing medical competence is the establishment of so-called perspiration or hyperhidrosis consultation times. Through the continued education and enlightenment of medical practitioners and also due to the new options in diagnosis and therapy, the treatment of hyperhidrosis has been substantially optimized in many countries so that isolated misdiagnoses and time-consuming wrong therapeutic approaches are increasingly excluded.

Acknowledgment

My thanks to everyone who, with their medical-practical support, whether by providing the pictures, specialized reports or publications, have enabled the revision, translation and improvement of the book for its 3rd edition.

My special thanks to the medical technicians and scientists named in the appendix to the book for their valuable collaboration.

But many of the sufferers and readers of the previous editions have also contributed substantially to the printing of this new edition through their constructive criticism, information and submitted material.

Hilter, January 2006
Dietmar Stattkus

Introduction

While even the smallest exertion, the slightest expenditure of energy or perception of warmth causes beads of sweat to roll on one person, the flow of perspiration on another person is almost entirely absent under completely identical conditions. One person will presumably sweat in the armpits, another on the feet and hands and yet another will perspire predominantly on the face or trunk. One of them is tormented, besides by increased secretion, by the unpleasant odor of perspiration which frequently accompanies such sweating, while another is protected against this secondary effect.

Sweating at summer temperatures upon physical exertion or intentionally induced in a sauna is tolerated as a normal phenomenon. Many people, however, perspire excessively in situations which actually involve no perceptible cause for outbreaks of sweating. Nevertheless, the sweat pours off such people in streams from the entire body or specific regions of the body. These burdensome instants are unexplainable for the victims. Their spontaneously appearing physical reaction appears irrational to them. They not infrequently sweat so heavily that they can no longer avoid the wondering and critical gaze of bystanders who are focused on this "abnormality" of the body. The consequence is a growing feeling of discomfort and being trapped, which in turn leads to an intensification of the perspiration. The phenomenon of sweating is then accompanied by a fear projected into the future of being given over to such perspiration outbreaks again in similar life situations.

The highly individually different forms of manifestation of perspiration clearly show that a highly complicated process is involved. Secretion proceeds abnormally and therefore pathologically, the transition from normal to excessive sweating being a fluid one.

A firm answer to this question is difficult to the extent that individually subjective attitudes of those affected decisively influence distinguishing between "normal" and "pathological" sweating. In particular, the psychological makeup of the person with the condition which lets him tolerate excessive perspiration but which may lead to deep frustration for another person, is relevant for the judgment of whether the sweating is perceived as a completely normal physical reaction or as a pathological symptom. Generally, however, one is justified in assuming that an unusually strong and nearly excessive sweat secretion, far exceeding its true physiological function, exceeds the tolerance threshold of the subject and is therefore classified as intolerable and pathological. In therapeutic practice, within the scope of diagnostics by clinical measuring procedures in some forms of hyperhidrosis the possibility exists of performing by standard methods a qualitative and quantitative determination of the sweat volume, permitting an objective assessment of the disease. In the event of an accurate diagnosis, this hyperfunction of the sweat gland is designated by the medical term **hyperhidrosis.**

The causes of the excessive perspiration are multifactorial since the disease may be manifested in the physical as well as in the psychological realm. In diagnostic practice this circumstance leads to many misunderstandings and unclarities regarding the clinical picture. The causes of hyperhidrosis cannot be classified as exclusively psychogenic or physiogenic. Therefore, the highest requirements are imposed on a well-founded and competent medical-psychological diagnosis.

A milestone for the treatment and diagnosis was the first classification of the clinical picture in 2004 in the 9th revision of the *International Statistical Classification of Diseases and Related Health Problems* (ICD), published by the World Health Organization (WHO), and especially the expanded inclusion of the diagnoses in the current 10th Revision of 2005. There the symptom patterns hyperhidrosis and bromhidrosis are classified with a diagnostic code. This international classification is highly relevant for questions of treatment, of the prevalence of hyperhidrosis, as well as for questions of research and insurance in the public health system.

The introductory statement to the pathological aspects of transpiration give a strong first impression of the intensity of suffering and the emotional pressure to which the sufferers are all too often irremediably exposed. But like the increased perspiration, the odor problem may also become a source of psychosocial torment for the victim. Pathological foul-smelling sweat is denoted by the technical medical term **bromhidrosis.** If hyperhidrosis occurs in combination with bromhidrosis, the suffering of the person so afflicted may increase immeasurably.

In the present book pathological perspiration is dealt with in two parts. While the causes and symptoms of hyperhidrosis are presented in the first part, in the second part a review of the presently most commonly applied and most effective therapeutic possibilities is given. The introductory presentation of the anatomic and physiological details of the sweat gland system is fundamental for the understanding of the disease and its treatment and occasionally requires the use of technical terminology.

In response to repeated request by patients, in the appendix of the book a review of the drugs used to treat hyperhidrosis and bromhidrosis is given.

First Part: Causes and phenomena

1. Function of perspiration

Under normal conditions our sweat gland produced about 1 liter of their salty secretion every day. During intensive physical work and under extraordinary stress our body is even capable of secreting up to 5 liters of liquid through the skin in one hour.

The two to four million predominantly eccrine [merocrine] sweat glands located in varying densities over the human skin surface are responsible for this. From the biomedical aspect the activity of these glands is a vitally necessary process that is indispensable for a person's health and contributes substantially to his well-being. The human organism is protected, to a certain extent, against life-threatening overheating by the process of regulated sweat secretion.

If our body temperature moves still within a physiologically normal range the secretion mechanism remains essentially inactive. The sweat glands intervene in a thermoregulating manner only when the temperature tolerance is exceeded by external heating factors or as a consequence of physical or mental stress. Cold is produced by the evaporation of the sweat on the skin surface, protecting the body against a dangerous heat buildup.

Basically everyone sweats, the degree and intensity of the transpiration being governed by a large number of internal and external factors.

1.1 Anatomy and physiology of the sweat glands

Anatomically considered, the sweat glands are glomiform [convoluted] structures surrounded by a tangle of nerve pathways and blood vessels. Channels extend from these dense glomiform glands as far as the executive organs of the sweat glands which are connected to the sweat pores on the skin surface and expel the sweat. The secretor part of the gland is functionally responsible for the secretion of the sweat.

The sweat gland cells as well as some of the secretory ducts are innervated by sympathic nerves and surrounded by smooth muscle cells, the so-called myoepithelial cells. Sweat production starts when these cells are stimulated by a sympathic stimulus.

The sweat gland ducts are approximately 2.3 millimeters long as was determined by electron-microscopic studies. The total length of all glandular ducts in the human body adds up to about 54 kilometers.

The sweat glands are generally considered to be the body's most highly functional glandular organs. Basically they secrete liquid at various intervals rather than a continual flow of sweat. A constant exchange of function occurs between the glands. Each gland has its own functioning rhythm, resulting in 5 to 13 secretion pulses by one sweat gland per minute.

Histologically and in terms of the material secreted the sweat glands are divided into two basic types. These are the eccrine and the apocrine sweat glands. The two types differ anatomically as well as physiologically.

The approximately two to four million **eccrine sweat glands** or free glands are fully functional in their total number from the time of birth over almost the entire skin surface. In neonates and infants the distribution of the glands is very dense because of the still small volume of the body. The eccrine glandular type has no relationship with the hair follicle or the apocrine glands.

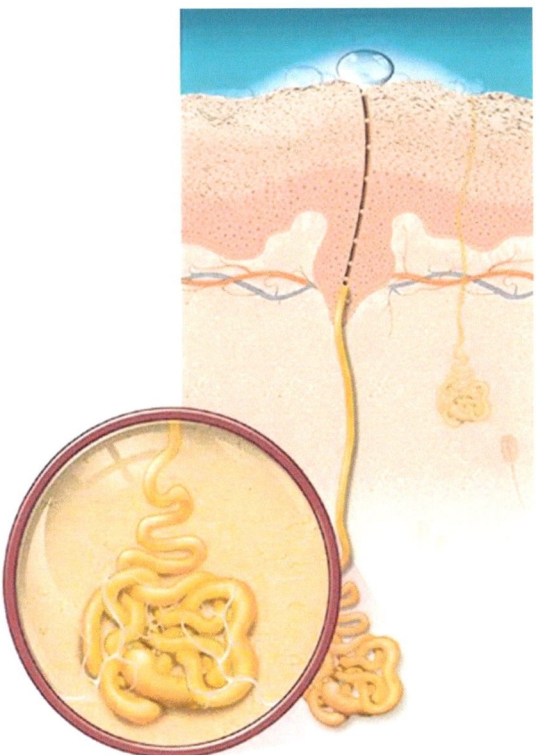

Fig. 1   Schematic representation of an eccrine sweat gland with glandular glomus (enlargement,) efferent duct and gland pore.

Eccrine sweat gland average 0.4 mm in size and originate in the epidermis. The are situated at the boundary between cutaneous and subcutaneous tissue. The eccrine sweat gland duct has it origin in the glandular glomus, straightens out and then passes over into a helical segment. This efferent duct passes through the epidermis and finally terminates in the sweat gland pore. The pores on the skin surface form the outlet channels for the secretion and therefore function as connection points between body and the external environment.

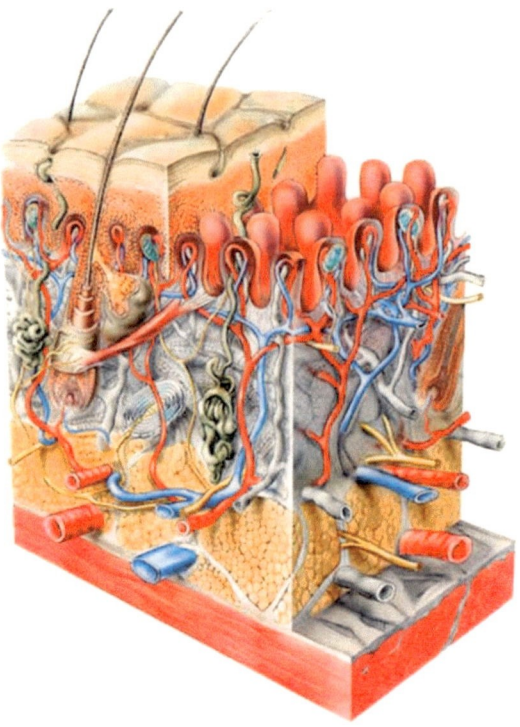

Fig. 2   Cross section of skin with eccrine sweat glands, blood vessels, hair roots and sebaceous glands.

The eccrine gland cells secrete sweat without damage to or loosening up of their cell structure. Their secretion contains scarcely any native cell plasma. In the literature the eccrine secretion is therefore frequently equated with the merocrine secretion.

Physiologically speaking, the eccrine sweat glands are responsible for thermoregulation as well as for the water and electrolyte balance of the body. The electrical conductance of the skin is also determined by its moistening by sweat, because the secreted sweat contains ions as good electrical conductors.

There are, on the average, 150 to 350 eccrine sweat glands on one square centimeter of skin. The density and number of eccrine glands in the skin are highly variable. The largest number of glands is found precisely on those regions of the body which are especially susceptible to hyperhidrosis: the palms of the hands and armpits as well as the soles of the feet.

Apocrine sweat glands are positioned predominantly in the genital and anal region, in the oral region and in the armpits. The apocrine sweat glands develop functionally only under the hormonal influence of sexual maturation, therefure during puberty. They are physiologically governed chiefly hormonally as a result of emotional stimuli.

The apocrine sweat glands, also called scent glands, excrete a secretion that is additionally enriched with cellular substances (cytoplasm) and thereby causes the characteristic and frequently unpleasant sweat odor. These large glomiform glands secrete a lipid-containing, milky clouded and alkaline fluid. Their relatively uninvestigated function is confined to odor-communicative processes and governs the social behavior of the person.

The apocrine glands have the peculiar feature that they stem from the hair follicles, as a result of which they are also predominantly situated in the body regions with hair. Their efferent duct therefore terminates not in the skin surface but rather in the hair follicles. Only rarely do apocrine gland ducts also terminate directly in the skin surface.

The secretor part of the apocrine sweat glands also consists of a glomus, the lowest segment of which extends into the subcutis. These glands may have a diameter of 3 to 5 millimeters.

A detailed anatomic examination of the sweat glands shows that the glands are connected to blood vessels and nerve pathways, but the nerve endings do not penetrate the sweat gland cells directly.

The eccrine glands are wrapped around with sympathicus nerve fibers which activate sweat production in the event of an autonomic reaction of the autonomic nervous system via so-called postganglionic cholinergic fibers.

Besides this, the glandular organs are strongly perfused with blood, a fact which fortifies the hypothesis that hormonal processes progressing via the blood circulation are the decisive factor for secretion. The well-known stress hormone, adrenalin [epinephrine] is responsible for a high activity of the sweat glands.

In the secretion process a distinction is made between adrenergic sweating and nervous or cholinergic sweating. In adrenergic transpiration the sweat glands are stimulated directly by the action of the hormone adrenalin.

Apocrine sweating is governed by circulating adrenalin and is primarily emotionally conditioned. It is influenced by factors such as stress, fear, pleasure and pain. Thermal effects usually have less influence on apocrine sweating. To this extent the apocrine sweat glands are not responsible for the heat and electrolyte balance in humans.

Nervous perspiration is regulated chiefly by nerve fibers of sympathic origin which almost exclusively innervate the eccrine sweat gland body. The most important transmitter substance and information service provider here is the chemical messenger substance acetylcholine; hence the designation cholinergic nerve fibers. The sympathic fibers are normally governed by the transmitter adrenalin. The cholinergic activation via acetylcholine, to this extent, represents an exceptional case in the secretion mechanism. The eccrine sweat glands react to thermal, emotional, and gustatory stimuli; in the last two cases the sweating is usually confined to certain areas of the skin.

The sweat gland cells display a secretion reaction both to adrenergic and also to cholinergic stimulants, but the adrenergic ones usually falls out to a lesser degree. The thermal secretion rate is higher by a multiple.

Since the sweat glands almost all react to sensory as well as emotional stimuli, it is understandable that mental stimuli, e.g., in a warm environment, can trigger excessive perspiration faster than at normal ambient temperature. It is also well known that emotional transpiring commences sooner than, for instance, thermal sweating.

The actual secretion mechanism is based on highly complex biochemical processes in the course of which the transport of electrolytes (especially sodium) is of functional significance. These electrolytes, however, are not secreted together with the secretion; they are reabsorbed before the actual secretion process so that there is no deficiency of these essential substances in the body.

The existence of another type of gland is also debated in the literature, which involves a "chimaera" or hybrid type of the eccrine and apocrine glands. These **apoeccrine sweat glands** are said to be located chiefly in the armpit region, which fact could also be confirmed by studies on patients with axillary hyperhidrosis. This third species of gland closely resembles the eccrine glands and under the influence of acetylcholine secretes many times more sweat than the eccrine gland.

1.2 Composition of sweat

The sweat glands secrete the most highly diluted secretion of the human body, sweat. This native fluid, which controls certain metabolic processes, consists of 99 to 99.7% water and only 0.3-1% solids. These substances are predominantly **electrolytes** which in aqueous solution are capable of conducting electric current. They include salts in addition to acids and bases. The distribution of these substances in the body forms a sensitive equilibrium that is called the electrolyte balance. Electrical neutrality exists in the body, because the numbers of anions and cations are in balance. The electrolyte balance can be dangerously upset by various diseases but also by athletics and work as well a under conditions of heat. The physiological process of sweating affects the ion concentration in the body. The water balance regulation functions via the ion transport and is closely linked to the electrolyte balance. In the case of extreme release of sweat the body loses some important electrolytes, primarily sodium. After strenuous athletic efforts therefore a thin film of salt is found on the skin. One liter of sweat may contain an average of 2.6 grams of salt. The secretion of electrolytes is frequently made externally visible by salt crusts on the clothing.

As explained above, depending on the type of gland producing the secretion, one distinguishes two types of sweat. **Eccrine sweat** is a relative thin-fluid and odor-neutral secretion. Eccrine sweat forms a hypotonic, slightly acid liquid (pH=4.5). The acid property of the sweat also explains the phenomenon of burning eyes when sweat comes in contact with the conjunctiva. **Apocrine sweat**, conversely, emits an odor. Especially in the armpit region one finds a mixed secretion, because both eccrine and apocrine glands are located here. Here the pH value is basic, in contrast with the skin zones where exclusively eccrine sweat occurs.

Half of the few constituents of sweat is composed of inorganic salts, the other hald of organic substances. The main component of sweat is "kitchen salt" ($NaCl$). The **inorganic substances** of the secretion include chiefly sodium, potassium, calcium, magnesium and phosphorus. Important constituents of sweat are also **trace elements** such as iron, copper, zinc and iodine.

The **organic substance group** of sweat includes urea, amino acids, ammonia, uric acid, creatine, creatinine, glucose and lactic acid.

After it emerges, the sweat becomes mixed with bacteria, dust or odor-producing substances which stem from the admixtures of sebum or due to bacterial decomposition of the sweat.

In the armpit sweat alone, besides water and salt, there are said to be up to 250 different substances present, some of them in traces, whose effect is largely unknown.

Just as the secretion of sweat is determined by individual factors, the composition and especially the electrolyte concentration of the sweat is subject to individual fluctuations. Thus, studies reveal different concentrations of the sweat liquid, depending on whether it is secreted, e.g. during exertion, in the resting state, when working, under thermal influence or after mental stimulation.

A great variety of substances are eliminated from the body through the sweat. This additional physiological function of sweat, which is called excretion, is therefore also one of the pathways of elimination in the **detoxification process of the body**. As an example, drugs can be eliminated via the sweat, whose active principles then also occur as an integrate of the sweat. Furthermore, toxic substances and waste products can be excreted with the sweat.

The composition of sweat liquid permits medicine to draw conclusions regarding possible diseases or physiological disturbances of the body. The analysis of the secretion is therefore used as a diagnostic aid and occupies a high position in medical diagnostic practice. Missing components or foreign substances present in the sweat may be an indicator of certain illnesses.

1.3 Protective shield against invaders

Human sweat, because of its substance composition, represents an important protective function for the body. Since sweat is continually being secreted over the skin surface, and man is therefore constantly sweating slightly even in the resting state, the **acid balance of the skin** is maintained in this way. This invisible release of sweat amounts to approximately 0.25 to 0.5 liters per day. Due to this acid effect, sweating has an immuno-dermatological significance in addition to its physiological function.

A hydrolipid film is present on the skin surface, an emulsion of water and fat. This film performs the defensive function of the skin and simultaneously makes it flexible. This protective shell consists of sebaceous gland grease and sloughed off keratin cells in addition to sweat.

Sweat leaches substances out of the skin that are necessary for maintaining the protective shield. These include amino acids, free fatty acids, pyrrolidone-carboxylic acid and acid metabolic products such as, among others, lactic acid. These substances are conveyed to the skin surface by transpiration.

The sum of all of these acid-forming substances results in the establishment of a relatively acid pH milieu on the skin surface. The organism is protected against bacterial infections by the acid film.

In the skin regions equipped primarily with eccrine sweat glands the pH value is about 5.2 to 5.5, therefore in the weakly acid range. On skin regions provided with mostly apocrine glands, conversely, a basic pH prevails. The sweat-related odor is enhanced by the basic skin reaction in these regions.

Besides the **acid-protective effect**, the scientists of the University of Thüringen (Germany) have found the antibiotic peptide dermicidin as a constituent of sweat. This protein is produced by the sweat gland cells and passes to the skin surface with the bodily secretion. It regulates the germ population of the skin and maintains its activity even in the acid and salty milieu of sweat. This natural antibiotic provides a long lasting protection against germ infections; according to scientists, the **antimicrobial effect** of dermicidin is one of the most effective protective barriers of the skin.

1.4 The sweat gland as climate control

A continuous release of moisture takes place through the skin which under normal conditions proceeds via the sweat glands as well as the so called skin breathing [respiration] of the body.

Human body temperature should be kept constant at 37°C independently of varying external conditions. However, the body is heated up by heavy labor, heat, thick clothing or emotional excitation. This causes deviations from the ideal body temperature which may lead to disturbances in the body. If no countermeasures are employed, heat death occurs in humans at a body temperature of 41°C, shivering at approximately 36°C, and at a body temperature of approximately 30°C already loss of consciousness due to cold. To prevent problems from overheating, the human skin assumes the function of an air conditioner.

Therefore, sweating involves a completely natural process of body temperature regulation. This regulation system includes, besides sweat secretion, also the so-called vasodilatation, the expansion of the blood vessels.

Measures for adjusting the body temperature are also called "regulating variables" in thermophysiology. Conversely, the organs or glands responsible for activation of these processes, are characterized as "final control elements."

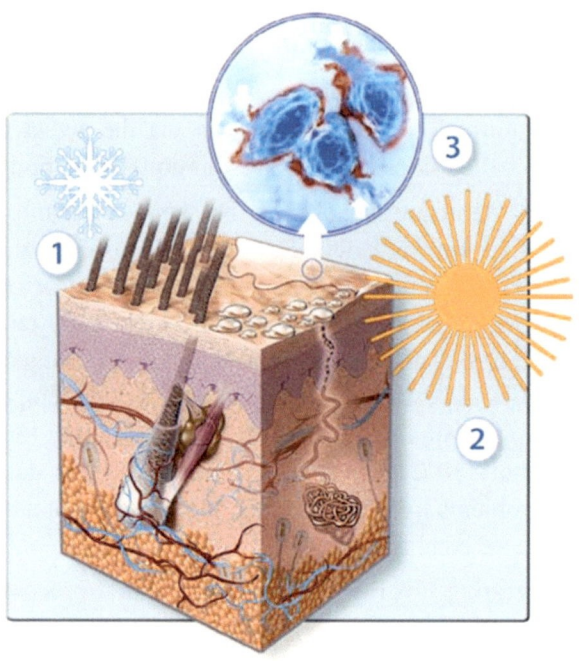

Fig. 3   Protective functions of the skin, environmental factors, variable temperatures, exposure to cold [1] and sunlight [2] leading to sweat production
(sweat area with metabolic products of bacteria [3].)

The different regulating variables are governed by neuronal routes,
the somatomotor and sympathic nervous systems, in particular,
modulating the thermosystem function.   The regulating variable
sweat secretion is governed in this case primarily by sympathic
nerve fibers.

The information processing and temperature regulation proceeds
via the hypothalamus, a part of the mid-brain [mesencephalon]. The
latter, as a central sensor, forms the integration center of the
thermoregulation system.

So-called thermoafferent nerve pathways extend from the skin through switching stations to the central nervous system. This pathways are linked to the peripheral thermoreceptors in the skin. Of these receptors, there is one type for cold and one for heat In the temperature regulation circuit the receptors in the skin or in the organs perform a measuring and reporting function; therefore they serve as measuring elements. They have the sole task of detecting temperature differences and passing them on to the mesencephalon.

The temperatures registered by the receptors are passed on to the final control elements for the purpose of actuating the regulating variables that are responsible for the temperature equalization. Therefore, in the event of an external temperature rise, the regulating variable sweat secretion is activated via the final control element sweat glands with the regulating goal of cooling the body.

Beside afferent temperature reporting, **efferent temperature reporting** also exists. The latter includes coarsely outlined first of all the stimulation of neurons of the cerebral cortex, which then pass information on to the hypothalamus, which in turn, when necessary, stimulates the sympathic ganglia via the spinal cord. These nerve strings then in turn activate the sweat glands.

The origin of sweat gland secretion via the efferent route therefore lies in the perception of the stimulus of the cerebral cortex, for simplicity the cortex. The route of the **afferent transpiration**, conversely, passes through the thermoafferent nerve pathways to the brain.

If differences from the ideal body core temperature are perceived, then the central nervous system, informed via the mid-brain, initiates counterregulation. The nervous system then influences first the bodily circulation. Upon exposure to elevated temperature initially the arteries in the skin dilate. As a result more blood can flow through the pathways with the effect that heat is emitted outwardly. This also explains the observation that many people display red and very warm skin in stressful situations or under the influence of heat, due to increased skin perfusion. On the other hand, in the case of exposure to cold, this system function precisely in the opposite way.

However, if the ideal temperature of the body is not successfully maintained, additional regulating mechanisms are needed.

Now the secretion of sweat is activated. This sweat is warm because of the elevated arterial perfusion (cutaneous hyperemia) and thereby differs from the cold sweat, which, e.g., is secreted as a symptom of a state of physical shock or as fear sweat.

The body temperature is lowered to below the neutral temperature of the skin by the evaporation of the sweat. This temperature state is then communicated further to the switchboard in the brain so that the secretion can be halted, because the perspiration process has compensated for the influx of heat.

Due to a dynamic sensitivity of the thermoreceptors, in the event of a rapid change in temperature, strong thermoregulatory reactions occur which subside after a short time.

The regulatory mechanisms such as in increase in heat generation by the body or sweat secretion are always in a state of readiness and come into play within seconds upon exposure to a thermal load. This also makes the phenomenon of initially extreme sweating understandable that occurs when one enters rooms with high temperatures from a place with a normal ambient temperature. In most people in such an environment a tremendous outburst of sweating occurs; this sweating is excessive in order to protect the body against overheating. This process is the so-called acclimatization. The human organism thereby quickly adapts to the excessively high external temperature.

Sweating as well as shivering are unpleasant for the human subject so that the person thus affected will initially attempt through appropriate behavior to take over the task of the thermoregulatory system himself by, e.g., fanning himself with cold air, rubbing his hold hands together or putting on warmer clothing.

It is striking that a large number of highly trained athletes have an elevated sweat secretion rate. This phenomenon can be explained by the fact that peak performance athletes have made a physiological adaptation. The secretion begins at a lower than usual body temperature. The threshold for triggering the regulation mechanism is shifted toward lower values; therefore, the athlete sweats relatively quickly. This phenomenon is also closely linked to the electrolyte balance of the body on which higher requirements than normally customary are imposed in high performance athletes.

Another form of tolerance adaptation is the phenomenon that residents of tropical regions sweat less intensively. Here the perspiration threshold is shifted toward higher nominal or ideal temperatures with the result that the tolerance range in which the human organism can manage without activity of the sweat glands is much larger.

The cooling of the body by evaporation of the sweat liquid is the essential economic function of thermal sweat secretion. Besides this, hormonal and emotional factors also influence body temperature and sweat secretion.

In connection with thermoregulation of the body, excessive sweating in the case of strong mental stress is rather a paradoxical reaction which, however, makes the necessary distinctions into emotional and thermal, healthy and unhealthy sweating understandable. In other words if excessive sweating occurs when the sweat runs copiously on the palms, soles, and armpits, occasionally also on other parts of the body such as the forehead or bridge of the nose without a recognizable cause, the economy of the transpiration is deficient. The sweating now seems unexplainable, unphysiological and assumes pathological forms.

1.5 The autonomic nervous system

The cause of excessive sweating is frequently hyperactivity of the sympathic nervous system with functional disturbance of the eccrine sweat glands. This fact necessitates a more detailed discussion of the function of the autonomic nervous system.

The primary task of the "autonomic nervous system" is to maintain the internal equilibrium, which is referred to as **homeostasis** in technical language, and to regulate all function mechanisms of the body even under altered environmental conditions.

As may already be deduced from the term "autonomic nervous system" these activities are processes which evade human conscious awareness. The processes of this nervous system take place autonomously with involving the higher brain centers, therefore without voluntary control.

The nervous system is controlled from the hypothalamus and the brain stem. Besides the hypothalamus other levels of the brain are responsible for controlling sweat secretion. Here one may mention, in particulary, the limbic system, which is purportedly responsible for emotional perspiration. Observations and impressions are processed and provided with emotional content in the limbic system. However, it does not act directly on sweat secretion but rather activates it indirectly via the hypothalamus.

The autonomic nervous system is divided anatomically and functionally into two systems: the sympathic and parasympathic nervous systems.

In interaction these partial system coordinate the activities of the internal organs and glands and thereby perform a regulatory function, primarily by triggering ultrafine biochemical processes.

Nerve fibers of the sympathicus and parasympathicus run to the internal organs and glands. The effects of these two partial nervous systems run in opposite directions and are therefore described as antagonistic. The common feature of these antagonists is the fact that from them nerve fibers branch to the successor organs or glands, and the systems are capable, via these nerve fibers, of activating or deactivating these organs – usually through their musculature. The two systems are closely coupled to the spinal medulla and the human brain, from which they get information about necessary control processes.

The **sympathicus** is primarily responsible for the activation of the organs, which is necessary especially in the case of bodily activation. It enhances the performance of the body. In the case of circulatory activity the function of the sympathicus raises the total physical capacity, increases the heart rate, the blood pressure climbs, the respiration through the lungs speeded up, and the sweat glands are activated.

The information is transmitted by the nerve fibers to the successor organs or glands within the autonomic nervous system.

The transmitter substance of parasympathic nerves is acetylcholine, transmitter substances of the sympathic nerves are epinephrine and norepinephrine.

Sympathic nerve fibers are responsible for sweat secretion. These fibers branch out postganglionically to the glands via a boundary fiber, the ganglion chain, positioned on the left and right sides of the spinal cord.

The sweat gland represents an exception in this connection, because, as opposed to other postganglionic sympathic fibers, it is stimulated cholinergically with the messenger substance acetylcholine. On the other hand, fibers of the sympathicus, in which epinephrine and norepinephrine serve as information transmitters, are called adrenergic.

The performance capacity of the sympathic nervous system becomes especially clear precisely in situations of alarm and panic. At the same time, however, the sympathicus also acts inhibitorily on those organs that are primarily governed by the parasympathicus. This includes organ activities of the digestive tract, the elimination organs and sex organs. The activity of the parasympathicus takes place in the state of physical rest.

The nervous systems perform their tasks as antagonists by mutually influencing each other. If the sympathicus comes into action, it blocks the organs stimulated by the parasympathicus. Conversely, the organs stimulated by the sympathicus are inhibited when the parasympathicus is active. Thus a cycle of mutual influencing is established.

The autonomic nervous system also interacts with the endocrine gland system of the human body. The latter deals with the body's internal secretion processes which exert an effect on the complex processes of sweat secretion.

The endocrine system consists of a chain of glands that produce **hormones** and maintain the hormone balance of the body. Hormones are substances that regulate the activity of internal organs and put the body into a state of alarm, e.g., in situations arousing fear, in the same manner as occurs due to the function of the autonomic nervous system.

The cause of psychoautonomic or functional disturbances of the body that are not traceable exclusively to organic factors may be of mental/psychological origin.

In these disturbances the interplay of the autonomic nervous systems is uncompensated, the interaction of sympathicus and parasympathicus is impaired. The disturbances are of variable nature in such cases and depend on the type of organ to which the disturbance is transmitted.

A causative factor in the phenomenon of abnormal sweating is a hyperfunctioning of the autonomic nervous system in the form of overstimulation of the neuronal transmission to the sweat glands. The causes of this derailment are unexplained, but emotional stresses, are demonstrably manifested on the autonomic and influence its regulatory processes.

The decisive facter, however, is not merely the intensity or the duration of the emotional stimulations; criteria such as the constitution of the body, physical overexertion, poor working conditions, hormonal disturbances, a fearful personality, or congenital metabolic disturbances play an exacerbating role in the evaluation of psychoautonomic disturbance phenomena and thereby also with respect to pathogenic perspiration.

2.   The symptomatology of hyperhidrosis

Hyperhidrosis as a clinical picture is characterized by secretion of extraordinarily large quantitis of liquid sweat. The secretion rate when hyperhidrosis is present is far in excess of that for normal thermoregulation.

Excessive sweat secretion in most cases occurs on the hands and feet, in the armpits or appears in a local combination. Besides this, however, the face, neck or the entire head of the subject may also be partially afflicted by hyperhidrosis. These locally confined symptoms in therapeutic practice are called **local hyperhidrosis.** On the other hand, if the entire body is afflicted by the hyperperspiration, one speaks of the presence of **generalized hyperhidrosis.**

Since every region of the body may be affected, the location of the hyperhidrosis is also accordingly multiple. Depending on the sweat centers involved one distinguishes the following locations.

- **Hands** (palmar hyperhidrosis/hyperhidrosis manuum)
  Palmar hyperhidrosis may range from unpleasant moistness of the hands to the point where beads of sweat drip from the hands, representing a particular problem in the everyday life of the victim.

- **Armpits** (axillary hyperhidrosis/hyperhidrosis axillaris)
  The production of sweat is usually triggered by situations of emotional/mental stress in which the armpits may become dripping wet and the liquid sometimes even runs down the body. In such cases frequently a pronounced and visible wetting of the clothing occurs.

- **Head and throat** (facial hyperhidrosis/hyperhidrosis facialis)
  In this case there is heavy sweating on the skin of the head with wetting of the hair and also in the forehead and facial region, which also can scarcely be concealed from the public.

- **Feet** (plantar hyperhidrosis/hyperhidrosis pedum)
  The feet may also display strong sweat production which, in the worst case, involves softening of the skin and occurrence of infections.

- **Trunk** (truncal hyperhidrosis)
  This isolated form of hyperhidrosis occurs relatively rarely.

- **Gustatory hyperhidrosis**
  Sweating, mostly in the region of the face, when eating often progresses symmetically.

Patients frequently complain of outbreaks of sweating occurring spontaneously within a very short time and unexpectedly and often differing in intensity and scope. In many persons who suffer, e.g., from hyperhidrosis of the hands and/or feet, a so-called palmoplantar hyperhidrosis (palmo = hands, plantar = feet) – the sweat just spills from these extremities. The skin surface of the body parts afflicted by the problem is therefore almost constantly covered with moisture, which may entail serious somatic as well as psychosocial consequences.

The determination of the provocation factor is used to classify a case of hyperhidrosis in addition to the intensity and localization. Thus, the hyperhidrosis may be of thermal or emotional origin, it may be provoked when taking nourishment, but also as a result of ingestion of toxic substances. The accurate knowledge of the stimulation of hyperhidrosis leads to therapeutic success more rapidly.

The different variants of hyperhidrosis can also be scored according to their intensity, thereby making it possible to distinguish physiological from pathological perspiration.

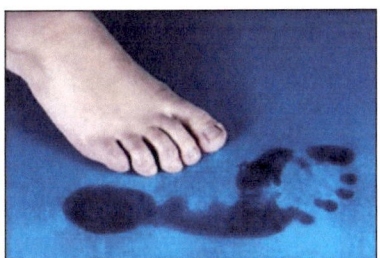 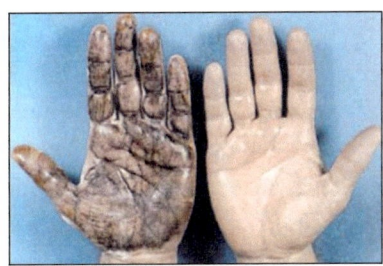

Fig. 4 Plantar hyperhidrosis (footprint on copy paper.) **Fig. 5** Palmar hyperhidrosis in the iodine-starch test procedure.

In the most common forms of hyperhidrosis, the severity is classified according to the guidelines of the German Dermatological Society and the Union of German Dermatologists as follows:

Classification of hyperhidrosis axillaris

Intensity degree I (mild hyperhidrosis)	The skin is only highly moist, spots of sweat on the clothing are 5–10 cm in diameter.
Degree II	Beads of sweat form on the skin, sweat spots measure 10–20 cm in diameter.
Degree III (severe hyperhidrosis)	Sweat drips off, sweat spots >20 cm.

Classification of hyperhidrosis palmoplantaris

Intensity degree I (mild hyperhidrosis)	Palms and soles are very moist.
Degree II (moderately severe hyperhidrosis)	Beads of sweat are formed, but the sweating is confined strictly to palms or soles.
Degree III (severe hyperhidrosis)	Beads of sweat form on the distal and dorsal surfaces of fingers or toes, as well as on the lateral edges of the feet, sweat drips off.

In the literature and in research there are different statements regarding the incidence of hyperhidrosis. In the US alone about 8 million people suffer from hyperhidrosis; this number was reported by dermatologists of St. Louis University within the scope of a prevalence study in August 2003. In the United States, 150,000 households were questioned regarding the occurrence of excessive or unusual sweating. The goal of the researchers was to determine the distribution of hyperhidrosis in the US population and assess the effects, especially of armpit sweat.

Of the calculated 7.8 million afflicted, 50.8% suffer from hyperhidrosis axillaris or excessive sweating in the armpits. The rate of distribution was significantly higher among the 25–65 year olds, thus essentially among the working population. Of those affected, 38% had consulted a doctor regarding their sweating problem. Women are much more inclined than men to discuss their symptoms with a specialist, 47.5% of the women, compared with 28.6% of the men.

Extrapolated to the world population one finds that more than 25 million people or 3% of the population are affected by this condition.

Hyperhidrosis has in the meanwhile become a generally recognized disease that is to be taken seriously. Rendering a diagnosis was facilitated by the inclusion of the disease syndrome in the *International Statistical Classification of Diseases and Related Health Problems* (ICD) published by the World Health Organization.

In Chapter 18 of the ICD under the section "Symptoms and abnormal clinical and laboratory findings not classified elsewhere," under No. R 61, hyperhidrosis is listed with the following classifications:

R 61   Hyperhidrosis
R 61.0   Circumscribed hyperhidrosis
R 61.1   Generalized hyperhidrosis
R 61.9   Unspecified hyperhidrosis
          Night sweat
          Excessive perspiration

Etiologically, a distinction is made in terms of the causes of the disease between **secondary hyperhidrosis** and **primary or idiopathic hyperhidrosis** in which fundamentally a functional disturbance of the eccrine sweat glands is present. The quantity of sweat secreted is clearly above the physiologically normal (normhidrosis) and exceeds the measure necessary for thermoregulation. Hyperhidrotics are frequently completely healthy people in whom hyperactivation of the autonomic nervous system is the cause of such a derailment.

In contrast with this, there also exists the phenomenon of hypohidrosis. This extremely rare pathological symptom causes the glands to produce almost no sweat, the consequences of which are far more harmful with regard to health than overproduction of sweat.

Before discussing primary and secondary hyperhidrosis and gustatory and psychogenic sweating, we shall first mention some forms of physiological hyperhidrosis having no real clinical value. Here, the sweating is due to exclusively physiological processes.

2.1 Physiological hyperhidrosis

Heavy sweating during physical exertion, athletic activity or in the case of thermal provocation is, as described, a completely normal physiological process. This relationship becomes especially clear when one resumes training after a rather long pause in athletics and observes with surprise how much sweat the body is able to produce.

Thermoregulatory sweat secretion is classified as a form of physiological hyperhidrosis requiring no therapeutic intervention as long as the regulatory processes of thermal balance are undisturbed An excessive and even extreme heat sweating, depending on the degree of the physical stress in question, can therefore be entirely normal inasmuch as that it serves to normalize the body temperature. However, if an imbalance arises here, the thermoregulatory sweating may also assume a pathological character.

A well-known form of physiological hyperhidrosis is **fever-related sweating**, triggered by fever-causing bacteria, the pyrogens. These pyrogens initiate a metabolic process in the hypothalamus, which raises the nominal value in the temperature center. If the fever rises, at first heat-producing countermeasures appear such as vasoconstriction and muscle trembling, since the body is initially too cold relative to the elevated nominal temperature. If the fever temperature then drops, the heat level of the body is too high relative to the ideal/nominal value, so that heat must be released by vasodilatation, skin erythema, and secretion of sweat.

Pain may also be the cause of increased physiological perspiration. In this case, nerve reflexes trigger the secretion. This is suggestive of, for instance, treatment by a dentist, where both fear and pain can serve as the sources of the sweating. Naturally, **fear-related adrenergic sweat secretion** also plays a decisive part here.

Withdrawal symptoms in cases of drug or alcohol abuse also have the physiological consequence of elevated secretion.

The consumption of **alcohol** is also a physiological process capable of leading to elevated secretion of sweat. Alcohol has the property of dilating the blood vessels and raising the base temperature of the body. This leads to increased perspiration, especially on the forehead.

Furthermore, the taking of certain **drugs/medications**, e.g., strong psychopharmaceuticals such as antidepressants, beta blocker or parasympathicomimetics may lead to outbreaks of sweating. In cases of drug-related sweating, a generalized hyperhidrosis is usually given. In the narrower sense, this involves a physiological process, but it may also be described as toxic hyperhidrosis.

Physiological hyperhidrosis may also be triggered by **inadequate acclimatization.** This involves deficient adaptation capacity of the body to spontaneously changing environmental conditions such as temperature and air humidity. If the body cannot adapt in steps to such changes, circulatory disturbances arise accompanied by outbreaks of sweating.

Some of the **phases of development** of man may also be accompanied by physiological hyperhidrosis. These stages of human maturity include, in particular, puberty, adolescence, and the profuse sweating of women during menopause.

The hormonal balance of the human body interacts closely with the clinical picture of hyperhidrosis.

From the standpoint of developmental psychology, **adolescence** is understood as an extremely difficult time for the subject, involving complex physiological and psychological changes, and especially also emotional demands and reorientations.

During this time interval the pubertal person acquires his final reproductive capacity; he reaches biological maturity. This phase is therefore linked to various changes in the body, which in turn may evoke emotional crises.

The hormonal restructurings related to sexual marking are predominantly responsible for the increased sweating during this period.

But the social maturity is also a desired goal of this phase in addition to physiological development goals. The subject is confronted with role and status problems in the course of social integration, which must be overcome and which frequently signify a great burden.

The process of becoming independent and the uneven paths of self-discovery during this time of crisis lead to demands which can quickly become insurmountable. Disturbances in this segment of life are often the trigger of diseases that frequently only become noticeable much later. Excessive perspiration, which should actually be temporary, may also occur in this phase and manifest as a neurotic symptom.

As a result of the development of secondary sexual characteristics during puberty the apocrine glands of the hair follicles undergo complete functional development. The production of odors typical of the glands accordingly does not appear until this phase. The sweat-related odor may become a tormenting psychological burden during puberty.

Apocrine sweating is also triggered primarily by emotional stimuli such as feelings of stress and fear, which frequently occur in puberty. These emotional factors are among the chief factors triggering primary hyperhidrosis. In the following, a special section is devoted to this topic.

Another developmental phase involving excessive perspiration is the menopause, called the **climacteric** in medical terminology. This phase of human development is viewed exclusively in connection with the female sex, so that this developmental stage is assigned a special position from the medical as well as from the psychological aspect.

The menopause is also accompanied by significant changes in the body which may in turn be triggers of psychological dissonance. The female body is adapted to a new period of time by the physiological readjustments, in which the possibility of pregnancy and reproduction no longer exists. Certain hormones lose their organic and sexually important function. The phase of menopause is necessarily linked to the cessation of menstruation.

The majority of women complain during this time of symptomatic problems such as sudden flashes of heat and uncontrolled outbreaks of sweating. These spontaneous hot flashes with sudded sweat outbreaks usually progress in a generalized manner, but a certain dominance of perspiration on the face and the scalp can often be discerned. This form of sweating is also called **menopausal hyperhidrosis**.

The symptoms of menopause are temporary. After the hormone balance of the woman has swung back to the normal state, the secretion of sweat will also return to the physiological norm.

The menopause is paralleled by many-sided psychosocial problems, causing an additional tendency toward emotional perspiration.

The close relationship between being **overweight** and a tendency toward increased sweating may also be considered as physiological hyperhidrosis. The subjects suffering from overweight or even obesity have a clearly lower tolerance threshold with respect to perspiration, so that the sweating mechanism is already set in motion even by a minor stimulus.

This context between adiposity and perspiration is also constantly especially emphasized and strengthened by cultural value estimations. In an age when slenderness is described as an ideal of life, the person plagued by obesity must deal, besides with physical problems, also with psychological difficulties whose source is frequently traced to definitions specific to the culture.

It is quite obvious that the body of a heavy person is challenged to perform more. Because of the increased metabolism, the circulation of a corpulent person is much more highly loaded than that of a person of normal weight.

The causes of the condition of being fat in the normal case are an increased calorie intake if no other disease is present. The human body requires nourishment to carry out its basal metabolism. If the food intake is higher than the daily requirement, however, this results in a weight increase.

The body can store and process certain constituents of the food such as proteins and carbohydrates only in certain quantities. The constituents of excessive eating are then stored in the fatty tissue.

The high metabolism simultaneously releases energy that is also emitted in the form of heat. This metabolism-related generation of heat leads to a higher body temperature, so that countermeasures such as heat reduction by perspiration must be taken. In so far, excessive sweating by overweight persons is nothing other than thermoregulation.

Moreover, the reduced heat emission due to the insulating layer of fat must also be compensated. This compensation is performed by the sweat glands.

A heavy person therefore usually sweats much faster and more copiously than a person of normal weight. Adiposity is a health risk and may be linked to adverse side effects for the person affected, including the tendency for rapid sweating.

2.2 Primary hyperhidrosis

The most common manifestation of pathological sweating is the form of the disease designated in the medical literature as "idiopathic," "primary," or "essential" hyperhidrosis. In such a case, sweating is an independent disease state without recognizable organic causes.

Such a paraphrase is used in medicine whenever organic defects cannot be found to explain a disease but the pattern of symptoms persists nevertheless.

The causes of primary hyperhidrosis are, for the most part, unexplained. It is a constitutionally conditioned hyperfunction of the eccrine glands at an elevated sympathicus level. It usually begins with the onset of puberty and may continue developing pathologically. The most prevalent forms of manifestation are hyperhidrosis of the armpits, the hands, and the feet. However, the trunk, head, and neck may also be affected by primary hyperhidrosis. These manifestation forms may occur both in isolation and in combination. In the latter case, one speaks of a combined hyperhidrosis.

In this form of primary hyperhidrosis, the sweat appears basically symmetrically on the predisposed areas of the skin and is stimulated by emotions, so that this common form is often described as emotional sweating. Thus, one often observes in the afflicted a quiescence of the hypersecretion during the sleep phase. Although emotionally provoked, primary hyperhidrosis involves a predominantly cholinergic form of sweating, in which the neurotransmitter acetylcholine is produced in excess. Especially in cases of primary hyperhidrosis. It is noteworthy that fear and stress factors essentially activate the sweat gland system.

The areas of the mid-brain responsible for controlling perspiration are in a close communicative contact with the emotion center of the brain. This center coordinates our emotional experience.

Because of this interplay, the person sweats not only in understandable situations, e.g., when engaged in physical exertion or when exposed to elevated external temperatures, but also when is under psychological pressure, when stressed or suffering from fear, such as in a test situation or when delivering as speech.

If such emotional stimuli increase in their intensity, when they act on the subject permanently, a pathological state may well come into play. The autonomic nervous system is then so overburdened and overactivated that it may initiate excessive perspiration due to the continual psychological pressure.

This elevated release of secretion is very embarrassing for the person in question. Self-consciousness and self-esteem are severely impaired by the increased sweating and the adverse psychosocial consequences.

2.3 Secondary hyperhidrosis

Secondary hyperhidrosis is a part of a complex clinical picture and itself has numerous layers. For the most part, it appears in generalized form and expands to the entire body. This form of pathological perspiration is a symptom concurrent with various organic and psychological disorders. In connection with this peculiarity one also speaks of the presence of **symptomatic hyperhidrosis** when the excessive perspiration belongs to the set of symptoms of a different disease. The perspiration is frequently the results of an infectious or metabolic disease. Endocrinological disturbances may also trigger symptomatic hyperhidrosis.

The thyroid gland disease **hyperthyrosis or hyperthyroidism** is one of the most common diseases that are accompanied by an extremely high sweat secretion. This disease involves a hyperfunction of the thyroid glandular organs, accompanied by a strongly increased secretion of hormones. Hyperthyroidism is often paralleled by hypertrophy of the gland, which is externally visible on the affected person as a so-called goiter. The pathologically high hormone level changes the thermal balance of the human body due to the accelerated metabolism. The eccrine sweat glands are activated by the increased heat productions. The affected person very easily suffers outbreaks of perspiration as a consequence of the hormonal derailment.

Hyperthyroidism is also a case of endocrinological functional disturbances, which refer to all disorders and unbalanced processes of the endocrine glands, which secrete their hormones directly into the bloodstream. Besides the thyroid, these include, among others, the adrenals, parts of the gonads and the pituitary. Dissonances of the endocrine processes may cause increased secretion by the sweat glands since the hormone system is interwoven with the sweat glands via the bloodstream. The hormonal effect on the sweat gland function has already been explained in the discussion of so-called adrenergic sweating.

Another disease that may have hyperhidrosis as a sequel is the relatively rare **adrenal cortex tumor** (pheochromocytoma). This hormone-producing tumor is a usually benign tumor ranging from a few millimeters to the size of a fist, consisting of adrenal medulla cells. Hormones of the adrenal medulla, epinephrine and norepinephrine, are secreted in excessive quantities due to the influence of the tumor, raise the blood pressure, and also promote sweat secretion.

A comparable organic cause of strong perspiration outbreaks is the so-called **carcinoid syndrome.** This involves a hormone disturbance related to mood fluctuations that are greatly exaggerated by nerve reactions and therefore typical of the disease. The primary factor here is a tumor in the digestive tract or in the liver, which is secreting excess amounts of hormones. Erythema (reddening) of the face and extreme outbreaks of sweating are symptoms accompanying this clinical picture.

Extraordinary sweat secretion can also be caused by **nervous diseases**, especially by injury or damage to certain nerve pathways (paraplegia). Inflammations of the brain (**encephalitis**) may also be the cause of elevated sweat secretion. Sporadically, hyperhidrosis may occur postoperatively, therefore **after brain surgery.** The occurrence of strong outbreaks of sweating is also not infrequent in cases of **diabetes** or **hypoglycemia.**

Anatomic factors such as exaggerated **size and shape of the sweat glands** may also be responsible for the pathological phenomenon of hyperhidrosis but only occur in rare cases.

Another form of pathological sweating is the phenomenon of heavy **night sweat.** If night sweat occurs for only a few days, there is no need for concern. However, if such a condition persists for a longer time, the cause should be determined, because night sweat occurs especially frequently in cases of tuberculosis or bronchial disease. Infectious diseases or an abscess with accumulation of pus may also be triggers of this phenomenon. Extreme forms of alcoholism also lead to generalized night sweat.

2.4 Gustatory perspiration

The striking outbreaks of sweating during eating are very hard to categorize. A special and localized form of excessive sweating tendency is the so-called taste sweating, which appears in connection with eating. **Gustatory stimuli,** such as chewing, biting, or tasting provokes excessive sweating in certain areas of the skin in the head-throat region. If sweating appears asymmetrically on the face, this may involve symptomatic hyperhidrosis. This is totally independent of the type of food consumed. It is triggered by any stimulus that causes salivation. It is not uncommon that the back of the neck and shoulder region are also involved in sweating.

Gustatory hyperhidrosis may also be triggered by **consumption of certain beverages or foods**, e.g., hot foods, hot spices, coffee, or chocolate. The latter occurs symmetrically distributed predominantly in the facial region on the forehead, cheeks, and upper lip. In such a case with a slight spreading, the gustatory hyperhidrosis is of physiological origin.

However, gustatory sweating may also occur as a **neurological disorder.** Then a segmental form of sweating on the skin of the cheeks is frequently observed. This clinical picture has also been described as the Frey syndrome or auriculotemporal syndrome.

In this case, the secretion of saliva provokes the activity of the sweat glands. This sweating tendency is frequently accompanied by reddening of the skin of the cheeks, by feelings of swelling, and not rarely also by a burning sensation when chewing.

This syndrome may be caused by infections or postoperative disturbances of the salivary gland. This clinical picture may arise as the result of a "short-circuiting" of fibers of the gustatory nerves with those of the sweat glands. The transmitter acetylcholine, which is common to both nerve fibers, may trigger hyperhidrosis via the pathologically modulated innervation. Then, if salivation is stimulated during eating, the sweat begins to run. The pathogenesis of this syndrome, however, to date has not been fully explained.

This form of hyperhidrosis may also appear after a **sympathicus blockade** (surgery on the nerve fibers) or within the context of **diseases of the central nervous system**.

2.5 Psychogenic perspiration

Scientific studies have revealed that strong emotional stresses promote the development of skin diseases.

With respect to hyperhidrosis, these results have brought to light the fact that causation may be almost 100% due to emotional factors. Therefore, excessive sweating often presents as a neurotic symptom due to excessive emotional pressure. Hyperhidrosis is then understood as an exclusively psychological disorder with an unambiguously psychosomatic course. One also speaks of the presence of a psychogenic hyperhidrosis.

In pathological sweating, it is precisely the human skin that occupies a psychosomatically outstanding position. Its symptoms frequently appear concurrently with emotional problems and have a graphic character. The skin, as a "mirror image of the soul," is a type of projection screen on which mental conflicts are displayed.

Psychosomatics encompasses in general the interrelationship between physical-organic and mental-emotional processes.

The emotional equilibrium of a person influences his physical well-being in just the same way as the physical constitution affects the emotional life. This phenomenon is not only important in connection with a disease, but can also be observed in everyday life.

Classic "psychosomatic" symptoms have found their place in verbal expressions: "He's a pain in the neck," "It gives me stomach ache" or "I get such a rotten feeling." With respect to the sweating problem the following formulations are used: "I've been sweating blood for them," "I was in a cold sweat about the matter" and "That really made me sweat."

However, if the interaction of body and soul occurs in an inharmonious and unbalanced manner, thus overemphasizing one of the integral levels of human existence, this may be the cause of a pathological state. Emotional conflicts may express themselves in physical symptoms, but a physical problem may also result in psychological symptoms, which is precisely exemplified by pathological sweating.

An emotional conflict is then no longer handled consciously. It manifests itself via a pattern of symptoms, which at first justifies the belief in an organic disease. For example, an authority or power conflict, a phobia or a diffuse fear may be the cause of the appearance of the symptoms.

Not every psychological stress manifesting at the physical level can be classified as a psychosomatic illness. Thus, one distinguishes between the phenomena of psychoneurosis, psychoautonomic disturbance, and real psychosomatic disease, whereby these are ultimately forms of disease that are extremely difficult to distinguish from each other. A psychoneurosis or psychoautonomic disorder is frequently the precursor of a psychosomatic disease.

A functional disturbance is chiefly responsible for hyperhidrosis. The symptom of sweating here becomes the primary burden for the person. From the medical-psychological point of view one will then speak of a **psychoautonomic disturbance**. A person affected by this disorder suffers especially intensively from the physical irritation. Although the sweating often assumes excessive dimensions, occurs for no reason, and is experienced as a panic-like state, no organic cause can be found, which usually puts the affected person into a phase of deep depression.

In the case of a psychosomatic disease in the narrower meaning, conversely, a real physical disease is present caused by a disturbed emotional life. Gastric ulcer is a textbook example of this. Such a set of symptoms does not exist in hyperhidrosis. Here, no organ or organ system is diseased. The sweat glands are fully functional and anatomically completely unimpaired. They are only excessively stimulated into activity.

In order to make the formation and effect of psychogenic hyperhidrosis more easily understandable, we shall now glance briefly into the theory of neurosis.

Neurosis in the broader meaning is an emotional illness whose origin is to be sought in the psychological and less in the organic realm. The content of the neurosis, whose causes are frequently in childhood, is a conflict between the ego and the ego-suppressed impulses, the instincts. The symptoms of such a neurosis often present themselves in the form of an organic symptom. For this reason, this form of illness of the mind must be carefully examined in connection with hyperhidrosis. The roots of the neurosis are mental unconscious conflicts between instinctive desires and tendencies and instinct barriers that impede their realization and satisfaction.

Since neurotic behavior is commonplace and at times even appears advisable, it is generally extremely difficult to differentiate between normal and pathological neurotic behavior. However, the assertion is true that a pathological neurosis is always present when the stressful state has become chronic for the subject and he/she remains totally ignorant of the relationships of his/her peculiar behavior. Since ultimately unconscious processes are responsible for this, the abnormality of the behavior is not understood by the subject.

Anyone who in certain life situations repeatedly suffers extreme perspiration, suffers attacks of perspiration regularly for reasons totally unexplainable for him/her and is greatly stressed as a result may by all means be neurotic.

Therefore, sweating may be a feature of an internal conflict whose driving force is discharged by the phenomenon of sweat secretion. The more often instinctive desires are suppressed, the more strongly marked the neurotic behavior ultimately is.

The neurosis may be characterized as an intra-personal dispute between conscious and unconscious tendencies. The neurotic conflict leads its own unconsciously dynamic existence in the mental sphere of the person. The repressed contents of the conflict, which due to their own dynamics create access to the consciousness again, are suppressed. This process is accompanied by unconscious fears. The neurotic person expends great energy in order not be exposed again to a direct confrontation with the contents of the conflict. The causal conflict remains unresolved and therefore continues to smoulder in the unconscious, from where it spreads its disturbing effects.

The energy invested in maintaining the neurosis is no longer available for performing essential life tasks, so that a neurotic person has considerable difficulty in adaptation and is frequently overburdened by the most commonplace and customary tasks of life, which is also frequently the case with hyperhidrotics.

A differential diagnosis between primary and psychogenic hyperhidrosis is extremely difficult since both phenomena do not have an organic basis.

2.6 Sweating as a genetic trait

Against the background of the question as to the causes of hyperhidrosis, we must also look into possible genetic aspects, which frequently pave the way for certain pathological phenomena.

Research concerning genetic sources of diseases has become a revolutionary factor in modern medicine from the point of view of biotechnology. The new fields of science human genetics and the special area of gene therapy are the main subjects of controversy, not only with regard to their benefit for society but also from ethical and religious points of view.

Hereditary factors have already been discovered for many diseases. A considerable number of diseases can already be classified today as exclusively genetically conditioned.

One frequently finds in the biographic history of a hyperhidrotic patient that family members are also plagued by the phenomenon of excessive perspiration. This is particularly true of primary hyperhidrosis. Since other carriers of such a sweat gland anomaly often occur in the hereditary line of a patient, the hypothesis that the phenomenon is traceable to a genetic disposition appears plausible.

Currently (2005), the University of California, Los Angeles (UCLA) is conducting a large-scale genetic study of persons suffering from palmar hyperhidrosis and their family members. By analysis of cell material from the subjects, the researchers hope to find more information on the location of the disease-causing gene, with the goal of finding new therapeutic approaches.

In the foreseeable future, perhaps a certain gene can be identified as the trigger of hyperhidrosis, but at present only the assertion can be upheld that excessive sweating may also be hereditary. There are also studies which confirm the fact that precursors of hyperhidrosis, such as an excessive predisposition to fear, may be inherited.

Genes that lead to a physical weakening curtail human freedom to a considerable extent. In extreme cases, excessive perspiration impedes participation in social life. In connection with the psychosocial evaluation of hyperhidrosis, the disturbing effect of such a set of symptoms is also especially pronounced in terms of lessening the quality of life of possibly genetically afflicted persons.

To be sure, we are not powerless in the face of such negative genes. We are not bound for a lifetime to a handicap as our physical fate. Productive forms of therapy exist, which may contribute to relieving such suffering.

3. Development and psychological support for hyperhidrosis

3.1 The typical path of suffering of the hyperhidrotic

The attitude of affected persons toward the phenomenon of excessive perspiration is decisive for their assessment of whether a pathological process is involved.

If, as a result of excessive perspiration, the relationship with oneself, one's fellow men, and occupational surroundings is disturbed, then the assumption is justified that a pathological state is present.

The fact that the affected persons begin to sweat extremely heavily in specific situations or generally have a very burdening effect on their state of mind. In the ideal case, they seek help, since these "derailments" seem increasingly unnatural to them. They turn to a medical helper with their health problems and corresponding expectations.

Before this happens, the affected persons are frequently expected by others in their social milieu to make a great effort and not to "carry on" this way. In such cases, it is forgotten that such "sweating episodes" are often symptoms of an illness not to be underestimated. At the same time, they may also be understood as a call for help.

A hyperhidrotic must often listen to numerous well-intended remarks, such as; "Sweating is healthy," "Sweating is the most normal thing in the world," etc. Explanations are often given, which attempt to rationalize the phenomenon of excessive perspiration, e.g., that hyperperspiration could be a concurrent symptom of other diseases (which may indeed be the case) or is a phenomenon that is related to other factors such as temperature or exertion.

These attempts at rationalization, however, are of short duration, because the permanent sweating incidents recurring without a valid explanation do not permit recognition of any logical relationship.

Since – usually primary – hyperhidrosis begins at puberty in very many cases, it is understandable that the question first asked is whether it involves a "real" disease or "only" a phenomenon occurring during this phase. Before juvenile hyperhidrotics consult a doctor, their social environment first extenuate or trivialize their condition. The symptoms are considered natural and trivialized. Thus, the true situation of suffering experienced is not recognized. As a consequence, the affected become socially isolated and often can no longer meet the challenges of everyday life. They are constantly preoccupied with their misery and only rarely talk about their problem out of shame. Their sweating becomes a taboo.

Then, if the phenomenon of excessive perspiration extends past puberty or – in the case of already adult persons – for a long period of time, the affected person is forced for the first time to consider that a disease may be the cause of this deregulation. The pressure of the afflicted in school, on the job, and in the family becomes unbearable. Finally, after a first consultation with a doctor, in most cases, the family doctor, the problem is approached from the classic medical perspective. This first consultation of the family doctor, who is confronted with this usually not unequivocally classifiable phenomenon, initiates the medical odyssey typical for a hyperhidrotic.

For the classic medical practitioner, on diagnosis of hyperhidrosis, the problem arises that the symptoms described by the patient are difficult to treat in therapeutic practice, and the syndrome occurs frequently in a scarcely measurable or spontaneously objectively perceptible manner. The practitioner will be tempted to discover organic causes. Immediate therapeutic aid can be provided if the sweating is actually caused by a basic disease, such as is the case with symptomatic hyperhidrosis.

Many patients have reported that doctors judge their condition to be completely natural, biochemically valuable, and therefore not pathological. Despite intensive physical and medical-technical studies, the doctor is usually unable to hold an organic deficiency responsible. In the absence of organic findings, there is consequently a serious threat that no therapy will be applied at all or that a makeshift diagnosis will be made.

Since the symptoms and perspiration attacks persist or even intensify due to psychosocial factors, the afflicted will consult the doctor again after a certain time. As a rule, this takes courage, since they do not wish to be considered fakers or hypochondriacs. Usually, the affected persons themselves or the therapist will now consult another doctor.

The fact that a doctor had already been consulted for the same complaint compels the current practitioner to initiate therapy. In the normal case, he will prescribe sweat-reducing drugs for the patient (antihidrotics,) in the worst case, psychopharmaceuticals, often with serious adverse side effects. Frequently, these drugs actually result in temporary disappearance of the symptoms. However, the symptoms soon recur even while on the medication, often even more intensive than before the drug therapy.

The patient, who now has stopped believing the attempts at reassurance, continues his path of suffering. After visiting the family doctor there usually follow consultations with internists, homeopaths, psychologists, and neurologists. A characteristic feature of the path of suffering of the patient is that the chain of attempted treatments is extremely tedious, and during this time he is usually given no help whatsoever or only very little. Self-doubt and a decline in self-esteem are thereby intensified.

Doctors frequently refer hyperhidrotics to psychiatric specialists. Referral to a psychiatrist is certainly justifiable within the scope of a clarifying diagnosis, but hyperhidrosis rarely fits into a psychiatric sickness pattern.

In the ideal case, the person suffering from sweating is referred to a specialist, a dermatologist, whose field of competence includes therapy for hyperhidrosis and from whom the patient acquires a certain understanding of his disease for the first time. A dermatologist specializes in the treatment and diagnosis of such disorders and will provide the patient for the first time in the course of his suffering with the certainty that a real disease is involved.

After the care and treatment deficiencies concerning excessive sweating and their serious consequences for the patients and their families were recognized, the number of doctors familiar with this disease has steadily grown. In the ideal case, a therapist, if he does not possess the necessary technical skills, will refer the patient to one of the seat consultancies that have been established in numerous university clinics and dermatological institutes in the larger cities.

It is also favorable if the doctor has additional training in psychology or psychotherapeutics. The differential diagnosis necessary will be more well founded, the more comprehensively both psychological and organic aspects are considered. There is no question that emotional/psychological factors may be important causes of hyperhidrosis.

Only when the patients know they are in the care of a competent helper is there the possibility of being freed of their disorder or of their suffering becoming more tolerable.

3.2 Psychosocial effects of hyperhidrosis – a vicious circle

Psychological conflicts may arise not only from the complex structure of relationships with other people in which persons affected by excessive perspiration find themselves but also from their own internal problems. Such an interactive process consisting of social and psychological factors is generally described as a psychosocial phenomenon which can have effects especially on the disease of hyperhidrosis.

The really burdensome aspect of sweating is that such a condition cannot be concealed as can many other diseases. Avoidance and concealment behavior is nevertheless commonplace and symptomatic for a hyperhidrotic. Every day the question arises of how and by what means to conceal the sweating.

In our modern society, above all, performance and success determine the social status of the individual. Humans are also guided by external conditions arising from their social situations. In order not to be out of the ordinary, they always try to conform to social expectations. Scarcely any room remains for weakness and illnesses. Because conspicuous features and abnormalities do not fit into the picture of a functioning society in which everyone individual must also constantly prove their efficiency.

Excessive perspiration is understood by outside observers as something contrary to nature, as a form of conspicuous behavior that is not "proper." Who will willingly shake the hand of a hyperhidrotic who's hands are covered with sweat? A sweat-drenched hand evokes in most people a feeling of disgust, often even with the result that they keep their distance from the person who sweats so profusely.

Visible sweat spots on the clothing and a wet or dripping head of hair also frequently cause the subject's fellow men to turn away from him. Persons plagued by sweating feel compelled to keep their suffering secret or to pass over it lightly.

The result is a permanent internal state of stress, because in a world where aesthetics, hygiene, and normality have high priority, there is neither room nor understanding for this type of suffering.

It is especially burdensome for hyperhidrotics when in interpersonal contact they are suddenly seized by an outbreak of perspiration and feel entirely at the mercy of such. One would prefer to avoid the gaze of one's fellow men, but often there is no possibility of doing so in the social setting.

Finally, for example, in a test, in a sales conference, at a meeting, or in a discussion with a supervisor, it is not so easy to escape, even if you would like very much to do so. Especially in the professional environment, hyperhidrotics feel the most handicapped by their conditions. This is primarily true of the contact and social professions where personal interactions are on the agenda. The result of excessive perspiration is also the impediment of personal career goals. The illness and its psychosocial effects stand in the way of professional advancement or even the choice of the profession itself.

In the hyderhidrosis consultation clinics cases are even known where the hyperhidrotics no longer consider themselves capable of practicing their profession correctly because of their unusually heavy perspiration and the professional problems it entails. Thus, hyperhidrosis of the hands causes major problems especially in occupations requiring fine handwork (e.g., watchmakers, electricians, opticians, draftsmen,) since wet hands make it almost impossible to handle the tools and materials.

Hyperhidrotic are strongly focused on themselves in overcoming their problem. They are consequently in conflict with themselves; attempts to consciously control themselves by demanding: "Now don't start sweating, what will the others think about you?"

However, it is precisely this self-consciousness that brings the cycle of sweating really into play. The afflicted thereby make the situation worse. Often they are caused to think of sweating by external factors, e.g., by a thermal stimulus or by an emotional burden, thus setting the whole procedure into motion. This triggering mechanism is usually not related to the subsequent physical expression of heavy perspiration.

The subject initially perceives a sensation of warmth at the beginning of the sweating process, chiefly on the body parts usually affected by the excessive secretion. He is afflicted by irritating sensations of heat and warmth, and these surges of heat may encompass the entire body. With the perception of warmth or heat symptomatic thoughts immediately arise which supply additional tinder to the stressful situation. The first flow of secretion follows.

The hyperhidrotic spontaneously searches for any possibilities and remedies for stopping the flow of sweat, but usually does not succeed.

Compelling themselves just not to sweat, the affected persons are then usually overwhelmed by an outbreak when they try most forcefully to avoid it. Especially when lucidity, concentration, quick-wittedness and self-assured appearance are required, the vicious circle frequently closes, and it is precisely in such life situations that the affected persons are entrapped in their torment. The person suffering excessively from the sweating feels physically handicapped, even worthless in many situations.

The result is that the hyperhidrotic enters into a pathophysiological process that is described in medicine as a circulus vitiosus. This automatic emotional cycle comprises the original fear of the afflicted, the process of sweating from fear, and finally, fear of sweating. The pathological sweating is constantly reinforced or maintained by this cycle.

Especially the social environment acts as an amplifier of fear, because sweating is nowadays predominantly defined as weakness and uncertainty. If in earlier times sweat was an indicator of exertion, performance, and hard work, conspicuous sweating today has a mainly negative image. Anyone who perspires excessively is soon stigmatized as a "chicken" or even as an unhygienic person. Therefore, a very great part of the fear is fear of being exposed to the "awful" symptom. The affected persons are consequently inclined to conceal their physical abnormality. This game of hide-and-seek has an intensifying effect on the development of the disease.

Hyperhidrotics whose hypersecretion extends to the armpits or head are especially tormented, because the physical hyperfunction can scarcely be concealed from the eyes of others.

Therefore, armpit "sweaters" often attempt to conceal the conspicuousness by folding/crossing their arms, because the obvious sweat marks in the textiles will then not be noticed. However, such behavior immediately triggers the opposite effect. The constant internal plea that no one will see "it" alone promotes a high secretion flow. The situation of suffering is manifested by this spiral of fear.

The situation is no different for hyperhidrosis of the hands, whose moistness and wetness the affected persons seek to conceal by keeping their hands in their pockets. This conscious behavior, however, intensifies the fear of sweating.

It is also very unpleasant for the hyperhidrotics who suffer to a considerable degree from sweating feet and sweat odor if the are requested in certain situation so take their shoes off. The mere idea of taking the shoes off has a demonstrably intensifying effect on the secretion process at the feet.

As will be shown in detail in the following, the clinical picture of hyperhidrosis may consist to a great part of fear, a fear which signifies an excessive burden, both physically and mentally, for the affected person, and therefore has lost its originally constructive, positive character.

Such negative, burdensome fear represents a reaction to situations in which the affected persons feel exposed to the reactions and criticism of their surroundings.

The hyperhidrotic is always accompanied by "catastrophic thoughts" such as: "What will I do if I start to sweat heavily again, what will the others think of me, they will certainly laugh at me..." Such imaginings are typical of this disease.

In social situations in which the affected person is exposed to evaluations by others, the fear flares up, which substantially influences the course, the intensity, and personal attitude toward the disease.

The subjects try their utmost to prevent a "disgrace" and make a good impression on the others. Since they not always succeed in this undertaking, a typical social stress conflict arises for the hyperhidrotics.

External evaluation is decisive for the experiencing of the disease, because the excessively sweating person believes that the attention of others is exclusively focused on his person and his abnormal "behavior."

The dread of a negative evaluation by others, the fear of pity and cynicism, coupled with the "effort" always mentally present just not to sweat, does not fit into the self-image of the affected person which is directed at social and physical functioning.

This self-image includes the manner in which one sees oneself, the self-perception, and tends to blank out negative aspects. The consequence is the manifestation of a stress conflict consisting of the elementary questions: "How do I want to be?" and "How am I perceived?"

Negative expectations and critical external evaluation also cause the affected person to suffer identity crises. The verdict of others: "That guy sweats very easily" is transformed in the inner world as: "I'm always sweating," "I'm going to sweat again."

The affected persons thus create an additional internal source of threat. A mind frame is created for what others expect of a person. Often fictitious expectations without any relation to reality are internalized. The fear of being exposed results from the conflict between external evaluation, self-esteem, and, of course, from experience with earlier evaluation processes.

The persons suffering from excessive perspiration may construct a great number of expectations in their imagination. They will act as self-assured as possible in their social milieu and simultaneously look for flaws in their personality that counteract an attitude of naturalness. In this search they will naturally find something, so that they are soon subjected to increased self-consciousness and negative self-perception, which lead them to suspect danger in many life situations.

Fearful expectations and intensified actual or assumed negative judgments by others then provoke the outbreak of perspiration increasingly faster and repeatedly.

3.3   Fear as the emotional cause of perspiration

Emotions and feelings such as fear, stress, nervousness, panic, oppression, and psychological excitation have a definite influence on a hyperhidrotic. Above all, fear and stress are causative for the clinical picture, an inseparable and complementary relationship existing between these phenomena. The two factors frequently overlap and are therefore difficult to distinguish from each other. Stress is often concurrent with fears; likewise a fear situation also signifies stress for the person so afflicted.

Stress includes an individual reaction of the person to determinants defined as stress initiators or, more commonly, as stressors. That fear therefore represents an important stress factor is obvious.

Stress is basically experienced subjectively, as is fear. What one person defines and experiences as a stressor may be experienced quite differently by another. What, for one person, is fun, merriment or even relaxation, for another, may be an extreme burden that can evoke psychological and somatic disorders and reactions. Here there are distinct parallels with individual evaluation of excessive perspiration.

Stress puts the human organism into a state of alertness and alarm, into a state of excitation, which, if it persists too long, passes into a state of exhaustion. If stress becomes the permanent state for our body, becomes chronic stress, then we have the foundation for a disease. The autonomic malfunction related to stress may cause the body to suffer as well.

Fear always also means stress, since nearly identical hormonal and physiological processes are taking place in the body.

Sweating is very frequently a symptom of fear. The expression "sweating with fear" is a commonly used expression, because the physical manifestation of perspiration is frequently the significant consequence of the emotional experience of fear.

There are people who, for the slightest reason, enter into a state of fear or its enhanced form, panic. When confronted with the fear-triggering stimulus, e.g., an encounter with the supervisor, the affected persons are overcome by fear symptoms, their heart begins to race, their respiration is accelerated, and they suddenly begin to sweat.

Other people, in contrast, are far from being overcome by fear, let alone falling into panic, in such situations. However, these people also have their individual fears. For example, they dread making an extemporaneous speech in a large auditorium or intimate contact with a partner.

The assortment of fears is almost inexhaustible in our modern era. Fears are demonstrably dependent on social and technological developments, which explains their constantly new forms and symptoms. The diversity of fears also clearly underscores their uniqueness and subjectivity. Since emotional sweating is a product of the psychological dealing with fear situations, the complex event of fear will be deciphered in a little more detail in the following: In so doing, we make no claim to performing an accurate neurophysiological analysis; rather the explanations are intended only to provide better understanding of evolving fear situations.

Fear is a feeling, a subjective perception that arises from a previously experienced stimulus. It is experienced as a threat to the personal integrity and therefore requires certain reactions on the part of the person confronted with fear.

The findings of fear research show that basically everyone, consciously or unconsciously, suffers from fears. The human susceptibility to fear as a prior condition for the development of fears of all kinds is individually subjective and largely dependent on the personality type of the individual.

Certain character traits, is a person rather labile or stable, introverted or extroverted, allow making a pronouncement regarding potential susceptibility to fear. A demonstrable regular relationship exists between these personality features and the individual inclination to experience fear. Thus, the labile-introverted person is much more susceptible to fear than the stable-extroverted person.

One generally distinguishes between innate fears and those imprinted by the processes of learning and experience in the course of life of the person.

The innate fears in particular have a practical and constructive function for the human life and its development. They protect human beings against and in danger situations and guard against injury.

Fear is therefore normal and useful, if a balance exists between the feeling and the objectively fear-arousing situation, the danger.

Fear always progresses according to a determined reaction scheme. First, there is a cognitive process of perception, the reception of the fear stimulus. After this perception phase follows the reaction phase, i.e., the subject reacts mentally or physically to the received stimulus.

The primary step of this sequence is therefore the input report of a danger to the central nervous system, the human brain. The danger information was previously registered by the sense organs and transmitted via the information path of the nerves.

Then, this information is processed into conscious awareness in the brain, a sort of decoding of the stimulus, involving an extremely complicated biochemical process. There, associations with the incoming information are formed, which means only that the newly arriving information and already stored information are matched against each other. It is checked whether such a stimulus has already been experienced and whether information relationships/connections are recognizable. If the input information is deciphered on the basis of an earlier experience as a danger, a fear emotion is triggered via the hypothalamus in association with the limbic system.

The hypothalamus is responsible for the emotional life experience of the person. The pituitary is located in that area, a gland which secretes a great variety of hormones into the bloodstream when stimulated. These hormones contribute to continuing the physiological stimulus-reaction sequence.

Governed by the hyperelevated hormone level in the blood, the adrenal cortex is also stimulated to secrete hormones. It produces the well-known stress hormone epinephrine. The organism is shifted by the hormone secretion into a state of readiness to fight or defend itself.

At the same time the autonomic nervous system is activated by the fear emotion triggered by the hypothalamus. Other functional-physiological sequences now put the body into a stressed state via the sympathicus as a part of the autonomic nervous system. At this time sweat secretion, among other things, is also increased as a classic sympathicus effect.

Enhanced performance by the body caused by a fear stimulus therefore makes additional physical-mental energies available for purposes of flight or fight (escape or attack.) These additional energies are a positive, useful aspect of fear.

If a distinct disproportion exists between the fear-triggering stimuli and the degree of the fear reaction, the fear loses its rational and constructive character and may have negative effects. Fear is abnormal if an excessive excitation is triggered as a result of a stimulus, and since there is no reason to release these excessive energies, the body nearly falls into a state of panic.

The experiencing of fear depends on the intensity of the fear-causing stimulus and the physical as well as psychological constitution of the subject involved. If the intensity of the fear is excessive and long lasting, this may result in a symbolic creation of symptoms. The excessive perspiration, like trembling of the extremities, is a striking reaction to fear-inducing situations.

The symptom of hyperperspiration, which may occur within seconds due to a situational or object-related stimulus, is a prime example of a reaction in panic attacks. Such recurrent intensive fear effects are then often the rood of psychosomatic diseases in the broader sense.

It is justified to ask why, in hyperhidrotics, fears, inasmuch as they are solely or partially responsible for excessive sweating, are, almost without exception, physically expressed by sweating. The answer is that every person has a so-called reaction-typical organ that acts as a sort of lightning rod in the case of fear-induced overexcitation.

States of fear may thus become manifest in the form of a stomach ache, elevated blood pressure, headache or even a functional disturbance of the sweat glands, as in the case of hyperhidrotics. However, in hyperhidrotics, one will also frequently find the tendency for increased reddening [erythema] and trembling in stress and fear situations. This underscores the assumption that an autonomic disorder is responsible for these symptoms.

Fear mobilizes additional energies that are not "used up" and which express themselves through the reaction-typical organs. The fear is then negative and harmful in its effect; in such cases, it may be the cause of or concurrent with an illness.

If the fear is chronic and if it is experienced with unusual intensity, then, as a rule, a neurotic fear is present which can somatize itself and thereby affect the function of the sweat glands. Neurotic fear influences the regulatory mechanism of the autonomic nervous system and leads to autonomic dysfunction, in hyperhidrotics to permanent excessive perspiration.

Besides fear-triggering situations, which indeed potentially involve a danger or stress to which the subject, however, reacts disproportionally strongly, irrational or unfounded fears also belong to the destructive phenomena of the fear problem. Such disabling irrational fears have developed in our performance-oriented society into a disease of modern civilization.

An irrational fear exists if there is objectively no danger situation but the subject still reacts with symptoms of fear. Many people suffering from pathological sweating will regularly find themselves in situations and moments overcome by perspiration attacks when there is absolutely no recognizable cause for such a physical reaction.

The subject then may justifiably ask why does the sweat secretion shift into high gear at this particular moment. Since fears in such situations are almost the only cause of hyperhidrosis, the unconscious process of the development of fear offers the explanation for the apparent "illogic" of such perspiration outbreaks, which seem to appear out of the blue.

For the most part, neither a thermal stimulus nor a physical exertion or acclimatization directly preceded the attack. Therefore, the assumption that emotional factors, such as anxiety and stress, are solely responsible for the sweat secretion seems more than justified, especially as regards possible therapeutic measures. The unconscious structure of fear makes hyperhidrosis incomprehensible to the affected person and difficult to analyze for specialist professionals.

As already pointed out in the discussion of neuroses, fears are suppressed from the consciousness, because their conscious experience would signify a threat for the person. The result is that fear contents are moved from the consciousness to the unconscious. However, there the fears lead their own dynamic existence; they penetrate back into the current state of awareness in response to certain stimuli or factors, and there trigger the above-described fear and panic situations.

Irrational fears and phobias, whose characteristics will be discussed in the following, are not innate but traceable to certain learning processes. Such a fear-learning process can be illustrated by the model of conditioning (according to Pavlov.)

Both classic conditioning and operant or instrumental conditioning stems from the explanatory models of behavioral psychology which assumes that human activity is governed by experience and learning processes. By means of conditioning the person learns to react differentially to vital processes; here one also speaks of the acquiring of habits that are important for leading a human life.

However, besides many habits that can be learned by conditioning and serve to simplify life, fears can also be conditioned.

Situations accompanied by highly unpleasant experiences evoke negative emotions. This reaction of experiencing negative feelings may, however, also occur in situations that are in a totally neutral context, in which, therefore, no unpleasant experience exists. For example, if a neutral stimulus is linked to a highly unpleasant experience, then a state of fear may become established; in this way, one learns to react to this neutral stimulus again with fear in the future.

Naturally, the process of conditioning depends on the intensity of the emotional stress. The higher and the more penetrating the emotional effect of an experience is, the stronger the degree of imprinting becomes, and with it the probability of conditioning. Often the linking together of natural and conditioned stimuli may already be sufficient in the case of great emotional intensity.

In this conditioning process, a natural, neutral stimulus is linked/associated with a fear stimulus, so that a conditioned reaction results. If the natural stimulus appears later in isolation, after successful conditioning, this is already sufficient to unleash the original fear reaction. After conditioning, the learned reaction may be triggered by other previously neutral stimuli related in type to the conditioned stimulus. This phenomenon is called the effect of generalizing.

Now, if a subject avoids situations with fear-inducing stimuli, then this leads to an intensification of the fear (see also the Cycle of Sweating.) The avoidance of the negative experience of fear is experienced as a reward, which additionally strengthens the fear.

We shall use an imaginary example to illustrate this model. There are many people who suffer from fear of authority. Thus, they already pass into a fear reaction when they are merely addressed by a person with authority, their boss, for example. Usually, a person in authority has negatively treated these subjects in the past with excessive strictness or criticism. Then these experiences, especially if they were very intensive or frequently repeated, have the effect of a persistent emotional burden and may have an imprinting effect. The subject is negatively conditioned to the stimulus "supervisor."

For example, if in the decisive original situations the subject displayed the fear reaction of blushing or heavy perspiration, then this reaction after the conditioning event may also be triggered by any other person of authority that he/she happens to encounter and even in a completely neutral context (generalizing effect.)

3.4 Social phobia

In the interpersonal sector, hyperhidrotics often suffer outbreaks of perspiration triggered by social fears, social phobias.

A social phobia is a special form of fear. The fear centers here on objects or situations with a social reference that objectively represent no danger at all. Nevertheless, a social phobic reacts with fear symptoms in certain situations. The social phobia, as a special type of phobia, may have many faces. It is expressed differently in individuals and is dependent on the personal experiences of the subject. Social phobias involve fear of other persons. The subjects dread being criticized, they fear that their personal weaknesses will be exposed. Since a direct social confrontation could make his weaknesses public, the subject very scared of this. Social phobia is very closely related to self-esteem and the self-image of the subject. Usually, the subject is strongly dependent on approval, acknowledgement and respect from other people.

Furthermore, a social phobia is fed by the above-discussed fantasies of catastrophe and anticipatory anxieties which may drive the person into a corner and literally into perspiration.

The everyday life of a person with a social phobia is determined by fears. As regards their self-esteem, the afflicted are dependent on the evaluations of others, dreading negative judgments so strongly that they imagine their own worthlessness. Therefore, it is precisely in human relations that the person suffering from a social phobia is most fearful. Such a fear structure is very frequently encountered in the personality of a hyperhidrotic.

It has been repeatedly stated by the so afflicted that, when the public is excluded and thus presumably critical gazes, they are only rarely plagued by their physical problems, which may doubtlessly be regarded as an indicator for the relevance of psychosocial factors in hyperhidrosis.

Fears and states of excitation in the hyperhidrotic run basically in parallel with the physiological symptom of perspiration. The affected persons perspire in certain social situations in their reaction-typical body regions.

Therefore, cognitive and emotional experiences are attached to the physical experience of the hyperhidrotic. These cognitive reactions include primarily the negative side effect that the subjects are no longer able to concentrate as soon as they suffer a sweating attack. They set up a type of thought barrier to prevent any cognitive function. Their thoughts are focused solely on their main problem, sweating.

These negative experiences of hyperhidrotics lead to another form of fear, secondary fear. They dread not only sweating itself but also the concurrent symptoms which, alas, are also revealed to the eyes of others.

The fear of sweating is a pathological fear reaction, whereby sweating is always in the foreground of this process. The fear itself is perceived in connection with the perspiration. The forced derailment and the revelation of the uncertainty in the social milieu are experienced as extremely threatening. Although the most urgent desire of the affected persons is to suppress their sweating, this wish can never be fulfilled.

The fears concurrent with hyperhidrosis are very quickly embedded in the memory of the subject; there they manifest their own dynamics and become increasingly more noticeable when the afflicted on the stage of social life is confronted with a specific stimulus. Existing fear contents may become enriched by new negative emotions, which make the pressure of suffering experienced more intense in the future.

Hyperhidrotics are stifled by their condition in their social functional capacity; the manifestation of their potential is limited; they are so inhibited that these experiences of fear even make them avoid any social confrontation.

4. Concurrent and secondary diseases of hyperhidrosis

4.1 Depressions

Heavy and unnatural sweating in those afflicted by hyperhidrosis often leads to physical and social bad feelings. The major psychosocial and physiological burdens are frequently accompanied by other pathological symptoms.

Besides the fear discussed above in its various manifestations, numerous negative emotions, such as shame, feeling miserable, or aggressiveness may be added to the clinical picture of hyperhidrosis. An autoaggressive reaction may also be triggered; the afflicted person feels terrible self-loathing, usually expressed verbally, for example, in the form of self-cynicism.

A very frequently occurring emotional/psychological sequela of hyperhidrosis is depression, which in turn may appear in multifaceted and complicated symptoms and be extremely difficult to detect diagnostically.

A depression, also frequently called melancholy, is a mood disorder occurring in parallel with psychoreactive but also physiological symptoms. Hyperhidrotics are frequently subjected to periods of deep sadness and moments of feeling unfortunate because of their pathological perspiration, which in turn trigger depressive phases.

Whoever is repeatedly plagued by tormenting and suddenly appearing outbursts of sweating, whoever feels they have exhausted all the resources for eliminating and controlling this suffering and is at the end of their tether is at risk of also succumbing to depression.

Low self-confidence, underestimation of their own capabilities, especially in social interaction, may be an indicator of depression and often leads to the depression-typical feelings of hate and disappointment toward oneself.

It seems easily understandable that hyperhidrotics are deeply ashamed of their uncontrollable outbursts of sweat secretion. The afflicted who begin to perspire suddenly and apparently without reason would prefer at such times to have the earth swallow them. If these tragic scenes recur, which is necessarily the case for hyperhidrotics, then these negative emotions are intensified.

The most burdensome feature of the sequela of depression is that the afflicted experience a double stress because of it. The hyperhidrotics are not only exposed to the stressor of exorbitant perspiration but they also see themselves confronted by a depression which, as proven neurophysiologically, is also perceived directly as stress.

Such a clinical picture, which as so-called concurrent depression is connected to a physical problem such as pathological perspiration, is designated as symptomatic depression. It is especially critical for the afflicted if acute depressions occur in connection with the perspiration episode and they threaten to become chronic.

Depression itself is accompanied by psychological irritations such as apathy, withdrawal from social contacts, feelings of unhappiness, helplessness, being overwhelmed, and melancholy. All of these emotional reactions can be demonstrated together and already associated with hyperhidrosis, but they become chronic as a result of the repeated occurrence of the outbreaks of perspiration; thus such a negative complex of feelings becomes the cause of a very difficult-to-treat depression.

The pathological state of depression is also closely linked to fears which often serve the subject as a "protective shield" against depression. The psychopathological state of depression may lurk behind the fears, so that therapists have great difficulty at first in diagnosing such a condition.

The depression, in turn, often entails physical symptoms, so that the hyperhidrotic continues to suffer not only from excessive perspiration but is also burdened with other organic problems, such as tachycardia, chest pain, respiratory problems, hypertension, etc.

In this context, it should be mentioned that depression may also be the primary cause of hyperhidrosis, because a depression very frequently occurs "hidden" and expresses itself through bodily symptoms. Then, the extreme perspiration is the result of the depression and no longer its cause. In this case, one speaks of a masked depression. A hyperhidrotic should therefore also consider the possibility of a depression as the cause of his unusual perspiration.

The symptomatic picture of the mood disorder – depression – is highly multifaceted, so that only experienced professionals can provide diagnosis and treatment. At any rate the afflicted should seek a differentiated diagnostic explanation for their condition that also takes the syndrome depression into account.

4.2 Diseases of the skin

Other secondary and concurrent symptoms of excessive perspiration may appear on the physical level in the form of skin diseases.

Hyperhidrotics have a constant degree of skin moisture on the affected parts the body because of their over-proportional sweat secretion. The skin of the afflicted is covered in many places or even over its entire surface with a permanent film of sweat, so that it is highly susceptible to colonization by bacteria, fungi, and other germs. Hyperhidrosis can therefore cause or promote skin diseases. Concurrent factors such as a buildup of sweat in skin folds, delayed evaporation of the sweat by textiles or shoes, and alkaline skin milieu for their part favor the development of such concurrent or secondary symptoms.

Hyperhidrotics who suffer from excessive sweating of the hands or feet are particularly affected by such skin disorders. These extremities, in the case of extreme secretions, are excessively drenched in sweat, so that the skin surface is softened and highly susceptible to attacks by fungi and bacteria. Due to this bacterial attack on the moist skin and especially due to contact with textiles, such as socks, severe itching and skin redness are caused; in many cases dermatosis are provoked. These sweat-related dermatosis are further potentiated by other promoting conditions, such as moisture and warm weather, as well as by certain diseases, e.g., obesity. Irritations and inflammatory skin alterations occur due to friction in the folds of the skin. Folds, such as in the anal and genital region or in the armpits where sweat evaporation is impeded, are especially affected. The high flow of sweat in these areas of the body may cause swelling of the keratin layer.

Especially in the case of sweaty feet, many subjects are additionally plagued by itching foot fungi [athlete's foot] or keratin defects. Bacteria find ideal conditions in the moist sweaty environment. The skin tissue in the interdigital spaces [between the toes] may become detached [peel off] due to constant contact with the sweat. This process, technically called maceration, results in stinging, burning, and painful skin peeling, often accompanied by an unpleasant odor.

Infections, such as eczema, blisters, or neurodermatitis, may be triggered as a consequence of excessive secretion.

It is nearly impossible to effectively treat these skin problems that are caused and maintained by the hyperhidrosis. At least a treatment promises no success as long as the causal phenomenon, hyperhidrosis, is not addressed and therapeutically limited.

Before discussing therapy for the various forms of hyperhidrosis in the second part of this book, we shall digress to the topic of perspiration odor and the possibilities of treating it, since this involves one of the most frequent side effects of hyperhidrosis. Perspiration odor may also assume an isolated pathological form, necessitating a special thematic discussion.

5. Digression: Bromhidrosis

5.1 The Phenomenon Bromhidrosis

The result of pronounced sweat secretion predominantly through the apocrine axillary sweat glands may be a penetrating perspiration odor. Such an odor phenomenon frequently occurs in association with an eccrine hyperhidrosis. The afflicted, as well as their social milieu, suffer greatly from this secondary manifestation of the disease. Social isolation at work and in leisure time, isolation, and severe impairment of self-esteem and subjective well-being may be the consequences of the odor problem. The afflicted often have to deal with concurrent psychological symptoms.

Perspiration odor occurs mainly as a secondary effect of heavy axillary hyperhidrosis and is defined as an independent entity – bromhidrosis (bromhidrosis freely translated means "stinking sweat".) Bromhidrosis is one of the most common diseases of the sweat glands.

In the *International Statistical Classification of Diseases and related Health Problems (ICD)*, besides hyperhidrosis, one also finds the diagnosis of bromhidrosis. It is defined explicitly in Section 12, Disease of the epidermis and dermis, in the subsection Diseases of the Skin appendages under Number L75.0, bromhidrosis.

The close relationship and the interrelationship between excessive perspiration in the form of eccrine hyperhidrosis and apocrine sweat odor have been established in clinical studies. According to them, approx. 85% of bromhidrotics also suffer from hyperhidrosis.

Bromhidrosis usually begins with the functional development of the apocrine glands in adolescence under the influence of the sex hormones and the onset of sexual maturity. It is manifest predominantly in the armpit region (axillary bromhidrosis,) where the concentration of apocrine sweat glands is highest, and may continue developing pathologically. The racially differing degrees of size and frequency of the apocrine sweat glands explains the phenomenon that people of black skin are affected by bromhidrosis more frequently than whites and eastern Asians only extremely rarely.

The cause of the odor formation is the decomposition of the apocrine sweat by bacteria on the skin surface and the liberation of the decomposition products, which result in the individual odor.

Apocrine sweat itself is completely odorless. Initially, the perspiration liquid on the skin surface has a totally neutral odor, as demonstrated by tests in which sweat was collected and studied under sterile conditions. Within a short time, however, bacterial decomposition products such as fatty acids and ammonia are brought forth, which then cause the musty-rancid, fecal, and sometimes even an acidic smell.

Further odoriferous substances of sweat, so-called pheromones, also develop. These substances are also decomposed bacterially, thus producing fatty acids, to which the olfactory sense reacts especially sensitively.

The odor stems essentially from the bacterial constellation of the skin. Thus, micrococci contribute to an acidic perspiration odor, while, e.g., lipophilic diphtheroids produce a pungent sweat odor.

Besides the most common for of axillary apocrine bromhidrosis, there also exists eccrine bromhidrosis, which occurs primarily on the feet. However, in a few cases, the hands or, especially in the case of obesity, other locally limited skin zones can also be affected.

As a result of the long-persisting and excessive moistening and swelling of the skin of the soles of the feet, the callosity or thick sole skin undergoes bacterial decomposition. This continual process of softening decomposes the horn-like substance, keratin, which is responsible for the stability and shape of the cells. The consequence is the subsequent formation of highly odoriferous substances on the feet (bromhyperhidrosis).

Body odor is essentially an extremely complex mixture of odors. It is not just the sweat glands that contribute to the typical odor of a person, but rather also the numerous physiological processes inside the body. Here, scents are accumulated that are eliminated through the skin with or without involvement of the sweat glands. This process is well known to anyone after eating certain foods and treats such as garlic, curry, alcohol or onions. Waste products and toxins are secreted with the eccrine sweat and contribute to odor formation. Drugs may also be eliminated through the sweat and are part of the odor pattern. Also, in cases of a disturbed amino acid metabolism, foul smelling sweat is frequently secreted.

This phenomenon of exogenous or metabolism-related eccrine bromhidrosis can also appear generalized over the skin surface.

The olfactory sense and the experiencing of smells are closely linked to the psychological perception. The perception of the scent of a person has very great significance for his interpersonal relationships. The olfactory sense is especially closely tied to erotic-sexual sensations and can therefore induce emotional reactions. Naturally, the experiencing of the odor of a person is subjective and individual, but nevertheless there are certain standards for classification of odors, which make the perception of an odor be a sympathic or antipathic experience.

People whose characteristic odor is experienced and defined by those surrounding them as more unsympathic, frequently encounter major social problems. These may even lead to feelings of discrimination, low self-esteem, or even self-hate due this physical expression. Consequently, they keep themselves at a distance socially and often fall into a depression.

Bromhidrotics suffer tremendously from the secondary psychological effects of the disease. The penetrating perspiration odor is usually (mis)understood by those around them as deficient hygiene. The afflicted are stigmatized and condemned as unclean, although they frequently bathe several times a day and use a lot of deodorant and perfume precisely because of their problem. The quality of life of the afflicted is quite considerably decreased by bromhidrosis. This concerns all areas of life, such as school, job, friendship, romance, family, or leisure activities. Social distance or isolation is the most serious consequence of the disease.

Suffering from odor is a form of martyrdom for the affected, since they must live with the feeling that their environment considers them unclean and extremely careless. This view is strengthened by the fact that many scents are perceived only by those around the afflicted, but not by themselves because of general odor adaptation.

The odor problem can have a psychological effect of causing phobic bromhidrosis or pseudobromhidrosis. The persons affected live in constant fear that they might smell bad, in their mind's eye they develop the notion of bad body odor and are finally convinced that they stink. A serious odor delusion may become established without the presence of any objective evidence, where the subjects tend to be obsessed with their own bodily appearance.

5.2 Treatment of bromhidrosis

What can be done to control bad body odor if you yourself or your fellows consider yourself a "stinker" in the truest sense of the word?

If a case of bromhidrosis is diagnosed, as in the case of therapy for hyperhidrosis, a dermatologist should be consulted. In most cases, the latter will have made the initial diagnosis anyway. Organic findings that may have caused a bad sweat odor should be identified or excluded in advance.

For example, the presence of genetically related metabolic disorders should be excluded by differential diagnostic methods. In cases of hereditary disorders of the amino acid metabolism, abnormally foul smelling sweat is secreted.

Well-known hereditary disorders that may be causal for a bad body odor include trimethylaminuria or phenylketonuria. Trimethylaminuria is an enzyme disorder, in which the trimethylamine produced by the metabolic process is not correctly transformed in the liver due to a missing enzyme, so that it is eliminated with the sweat and causes a fishlike odor (fish odor syndrome.) In phenylketonuria, a hereditary metabolic deficiency is present, in which the essential amino acid phenylalanine is not transformed, resulting in an accumulation of phenylalanine in the blood. Since part of the phenylalanine is now transformed into phenylpyruvic acid via a different metabolic pathway, which is eliminated with the urine and sweat, the sweat will now have the smell of mouse feces typical for this disorder.

A disease of the armpit hair caused by bacteria (trichobacteriosis,) characterized by a superficial, usually whitish-yellow deposit of bacteria on the armpit or, in rare cases, pubic hair, may cause bromhidrosis and should be taken into account in a differential diagnosis.

The creation and strict observance of a program of body hygiene is an essential prior condition for the treatment and prevention of bromhidrosis. Bad odors can be prevented by washing regularly with an antibacterially active and skin-pH-preserving acid soap or scrubbing lotion and by using deodorants with a bacterial-flora-reducing effect. Frequent changing of socks and an appropriate choice of clothing and footwear are criteria to be considered together with the therapy.

One can often succeed in at least ameliorating the exogenously caused (food, medication) sweat odor by changing the diet, because bad eating habits may be the cause of the odor. Fresh foods low in roughage and high in vegetables should be on the diet menu of a bromhidrotic. Meat should be avoided, because eliminating protein compounds can reduce intensive odor.

To promote the therapy, the bromhidrotic should also avoid sweat-inducing treats such as alcohol, coffee or hot spices.

The therapy itself often begins with the internal and external application of fruit vinegar. Cider vinegar, for example, enhances normal sweat secretion by regulating the skin pH.

Apple cider vinegar is also beneficial to the metabolism and stimulates the expulsion of waste products and toxins from the skin. Fruit vinegar may be drunk and applied externally to the affected skin areas. Vinegar has a cooling and soothing effect on the skin and reduces the sweat odor when used as a whole-body wash or for hand and foot baths. It is also good for the armpits.

In cases of persistent bromhidrosis, it is necessary to remove the armpit hair in order to suppress the accumulation of sweat and bacteria on the hair stems. Apocrine glands secrete sweat into the hair follicles. If they are removed, the sweat is forced to evaporate faster and the odor problem is reduced.

There are various methods for removing the hair. After simple shaving, an alcohol solution should be applied for cleaning. In the case of laser depilation, the hair is removed by destroying the hair root, so the hairs only grow back again slowly.

The most effective method for removing hair in cases of bromhidrosis is electrolysis therapy. The hairs and the hair follicles are permanently destroyed in a painstaking and time-consuming process with electric current. This is a dermatological therapy procedure used primarily to treat axillary bromhidrosis. Additional information is available in dermatological or cosmetic clinics and institutes.

The antibacterial effect of aluminum chloride has proven highly effective when used against sweat odor, especially for treatment of the feet. The application of drying powders or sprays with zinc and talcum or tannic acids such as tannin may also reduce the bacterial flora in the affected skin areas.

There also now exist textiles with special chemical qualities that bind or even transform odor-causing substances. Even pieces of metal, algae and crystals are used to reduce odor. No scientific evidence is available concerning such procedures.

Besides conservative measures for relieving mild forms of bromhidrosis, the physical and surgical therapies discussed in the following chapters also come under consideration as treatment options. Especially in the case of pungent foot sweat odor, tap water iontophoresis is recommendable. In cases of axillary bromhidrosis, surgical procedures such as excision or liposuction of the sweat glands may also be given consideration.

5.3 Deodorants

Besides the antiperspirants as a means of controlling excessive sweat production, which are listed in the second part of the book, there are also preparations for deodorizing perspiration odor available on the market.

These are the so-called deodorants, which are sold as sprays, sticks, powders, soaps, or lotion. The essential difference between sweat-reducing antiperspirants and deodorizing products is that the latter are used chiefly for preventing as well as for eliminating or masking sweat odors. Sweat formation itself is not prevented by the application of a pure deodorant. Therefore, the deodorants are usually cosmetics, while antiperspirants are classified as drugs.

This distinction, however, is superficial, because increasingly combined preparations with both sweat-inhibiting and antibacterial, and therefore odor-reducing effects are on the market. Many deodorants today contain metal salts that contribute to an astringent effect.

By concealing the unpleasant and annoying body odor with a deodorant the subject experiences a high measure of security, which is important and desirable especially in social interaction.

The wide assortment on the market shows how significant deodorants are. The deodorizing substances can basically be classified into four groups. There are products which mainly cover body and sweat odor, those which inhibit odor by oxidizing odoriferous substances on the skin, others which suppress the odor by absorption, and those contributing to inhibition of the bacterial flora on the skin surface.

Substances that conceal or cover the odor are mainly essential oils. These oils mask the unpleasant odor of sweat and thereby contribute to the well-being of the user. The odor-accompanying skin perspiration can very easily be concealed by applying these agents.

On the other hand, oxidizing substances contain oxygen-containing compounds that react with the odor-producing substances on the skin surface and thereby contribute to reducing the odor. An odorless compound is created by binding to an oxygen atom. These oxidizing substances include the so-called peroxides.

The group of absorbing substances includes powder with a special binding capacity. Their effect is based on the fact that the odor-provoking substances are absorbed and thereby lose their odor intensity.

Deodorants that limit bacterial flora are substances with a germ-inhibiting action which degrade/decompose bacterial substances.

To support the function of deodorants in the case of heavy sweating, daily cleaning of certain skin areas, especially the armpits and genital region, is necessary.

As is known, by washing with normal soap and generally alkali-containing products one is intervening in the skin acid balance. Too frequent washing of the skin with such agents with a pH of 8–12 has an unfavorable effect on the skin's protective cover against acid. If this protective cover is removed by constant cleaning, the skin becomes susceptible to various pathogens. Therefore, the use of antibacterial , acid soaps is recommended.

When soaps and deodorants are used, the tolerance of the skin for the constituents is of importance. Soaps and deodorants are often triggers of allergic skin reactions. In the case of frequent use or of a special skin sensitivity, some components of deodorants may also cause eczema.

Second Part: Therapies

1. Therapy options in hyperhidrosis

While in the first part of the book the causes and symptoms of the clinical picture of hyperhidrosis were analyzed against the background of the multi-faceted and complex factors of influence, in the following, the question of possible forms of therapy, crucial to the afflicted, is discussed.

Due to the results obtained in recent years from research and medical theory regarding the function, provocation and blocking of the sweat glands, there now exists a wide and constantly updated spectrum of therapies for the treatment of the various forms of pathological perspiration. This assortment of treatments extends from topical therapy with sweat-inhibiting agents (external, locally limited therapy) through systemic therapy (internal therapy by taking medications,) physical therapy (current bath,) psychotherapy, and intradermal botulinum toxin injections, all the way to surgical interventions, such as endoscopic sympathicus blockade or curettage of the sweat glands (aspiration hidrectomy.) The effect of the therapeutic procedures can often be increased even further by their combination.

These therapeutic measures are based on different principles of action. The efferent ducts of the sweat glands are mechanically closed by local application of, e.g., metal salts or tannic acids. Conversely, systemic or topical application of anticholinergics inhibits the end transmission of the nerves to the sweat glands, while, in the case of tap water iontophoresis, the inhibition or functional closure of the glandular epithelium (theory) causes a sweat reduction. Sweat production is halted due to chemical denervation of the glands by injection of botulinum toxin. Surgical denervation or ganglion blockade is also the action mechanism of the surgical operations of sympathicolysis and sympathectomy, while, in the case of subcutaneous sweat gland suction curettage or excision of the local glandular field, the target organs (sweat glands) are removed. In the following, these procedures and their (neuro)physiological effects are described in more detail.

The therapies described will assure the afflicted that there is justified hope for a cure. This is also confirmed by the reports of former afflicted persons who successfully relieved their suffering therapeutically.

Which therapeutic procedure is ultimately applied for a given patient depends on the symptomatology and the severity of the hyperhidrosis. Treatment with creams or metal solutions, physical therapy, botox injection or surgery may be used. In cases of generalized hyperhidrosis, the treatment potential is currently still limited.

Basically, however, it can be shown from therapeutic practice that both generalized and localized hyperhidrosis are effectively treatable by application of the optional procedures and remedies now available.

Besides the factors of type and intensity of hyperhidrosis, the success of the therapy is also influenced by other components. In particular, individual tolerance for a therapeutic procedure; hence, the question of its potential side effects decides whether a treatment can succeed. However, the psychological status of the subject and not least the competence and experience of the therapist also play a central role in the efficacy of a form of therapy.

The results of the various therapies cannot be generalized, nor can their effect in the individual case be predicted. A maximal therapeutic result, however, will be related to the professional competence and level of knowledge of the practitioner.

Besides the above-mentioned therapeutic procedures, highly effective psychological interventions may also relieve hyperfunction of the sweat glands and may be employed in isolation and concurrently with other forms of therapy. It is precisely the psychologically active procedures, such as relaxation techniques, which provide support of particular value in the presence of emotional hyperhidrosis.

In dermatological therapy for hyperhidrosis, the application of a stepwise treatment is widely practiced. This is a causal therapy whose goal is to eliminate the disturbance responsible for the hyperhidrosis. An absolute prior condition for such treatment is the determination of any internal-medical, metabolic or neurological disturbances. When such basic diseases can be excluded, the further treatment is guided by a stepwise plan.

The knowledge of this stepwise therapy, which covers all known forms of hyperhidrosis and their healing methods, is of decisive importance both for the afflicted and also for the practitioners. Within the framework of the stepwise plan one first treats with the mildest remedies, which, in the event of failure, are replaced by the next therapeutically more intensive step. At the end of the therapy, in the case of persistent symptoms, there may even be a surgical operation.

2. Measures concurrent with therapy

The components which may accompany a successful therapy include consideration of factors that influence the flow of perspiration. The prophylactic measures presented above concerning bromhidrosis may also be applied in the presence of hyperhidrosis.

In particular, the fields of nutrition, clothing, hygiene and stress offer many approaches which, when properly considered, may contribute to a positive course of therapy. If certain habits are broken or new habits learned, the patient is making an effective contribution to controlling his perspiration.

Such concurrent measures may have a stabilizing and beneficial effect on the body in general and on the circulation, especially in the treatment of emotional hyperhidrosis.

2.1 Nutrition

It has already been pointed out that certain foods and treats, hot foods and beverages, strong spices, alcohol, tea and coffee stimulate secretion. This stimulus is especially significant in gustatory hyperhidrosis.

This involves predominantly normal physiological processes and relationships. Excessive consumption of tea, coffee, nicotine, or alcohol has a more or less activating effect on the perspiration balance of everyone, although this is not necessarily pathological.

Limitation or avoidance of "sweat-inducing" foods and treats has hardly any effect on a severe form of hyperhidrosis. However, an increased intensity of already high secretion can be demonstrably suppressed in this way.

Avoiding consumption may have a positive therapeutic effect and is presumably advantageous for the health. In the treatment of hyperhidrosis, a change in eating habits, however, results in a noteworthy amelioration only in the very mild forms of the disease.

2.2 Hygiene

Doctors and pharmacists often give advice on hygienic behavior to people with perspiration problems. The cleanliness routine undoubtedly belongs to the standard program of preventing perspiration and odor. The use of antiperspirants and deodorants reduces the secretion and frequently also the odor of sweat.

However, advising a hyperhidrotic whose hands and feet are afflicted by excessive sweating to wash them as often as possible, although well intended, is only of limited help. Hygiene is precisely usually not lacking in these patients. Quite the contrary, they usually wash, shower, and bathe much more frequently than other people. In the worst case, the constant washing may even give rise to a pathological cleaning compulsion. Very frequent showering or bathing is also detrimental to the protective layer against acid of the skin.

Hyperhidrosis is neither a hygienic nor a cosmetic problem. Good hygiene contributes only to the basic conditions of successful therapy.

2.3 Clothing

Wearing air-permeable and light clothing is also one possibility of therapy support. Respiration-active clothing from natural fibers should be preferred over synthetic textiles. This is especially true for all people suffering from sweaty feet. Here particular attention should be paid to the material of stockings and shoes.

It seems plausible that a hyperhidrotic should change socks frequently. This does not, to be sure, reduce the flow of secretion, but rather serves for hygiene and odor prevention.

Synthetic textiles may also have an intensifying effect on perspiration, but, above all, they promote sweat odor. Some synthetic textiles absorb the lipophilic substances of sweat, resulting in a penetrating sweat odor. Aside from the relationships described above, the clothing, provided that it conforms to the weather conditions and outdoor temperature, has no effect on pathological perspiration.

The medical cause of the sweating is not considered in the choice of clothing. Only the consequences of hyperperspiration, such as especially sweat odor, can be reduced by the correct choice of textiles.

2.4 Remedies without side effects

According to the results of a survey, hyperhidrosis in the armpit area is the most common and most distressing sweating disease.

Besides conventional medical therapy methods that may be accompanied by side effects, there are also natural cosmetic aids in the form of armpit pads that cling to the skin. These pads do not intervene in the natural process of sweating, but nevertheless may be effective in protecting against sweat spots and salt marks on the clothing.

These aids are respiration-active absorptive cushions with high wear comfort. Their main component is a high-quality, absorbent, soft nonwoven fabric which draws the sweat rapidly to the inside of the pad. The sweat is isolated and securely sequestered. Despite air and water vapor permeability, these absorptive pads are also highly effective against odor formation due to pathological sweating.

The pads are affixed to the shaved armpit region by a skin-compatible and securely adhering adhesive strip and provide security for several hours. They are especially suitable for socially relevant situations where the subjects wish to have dry armpits and freedom from odor.

This product is a natural therapy alternative for the person suffering from axillary hyperhidrosis and, depending on the situation, may be used rapidly, invisibly, and effectively to protect against perspiration and odor.

2.5 Household remedies

The use of plant substances is one of the low-side-effect concurrent therapy measures and usually comes under the heading of household remedies. These plant remedies – sage is probably one the best known sweat-reducing extracts – may bring about a reduction of perspiration in mild cases, but in the overwhelming majority of hyperhidrotics these remedies have only a slight ameliorating effect.

Also, bath applications with extracts of willow, oak, and maple bark are included among the traditional household remedies. The plant parts are boiled with water to form a decoction and added in portions to the bath water. Such a bath cure may have a sweat-reducing, astringent effect when applied repeatedly. No scientific evidence of the effect of such applications is available.

Another household remedy is potassium permanganate, which is available in drugstores. This is a mineral substance that is dissolved in water in a low concentration. Then, the hyperhidrotic skin zones are washed and rinsed with this solution. This process is also said to cause pronounced sweat reduction.

The so-called alternating shower is also frequently mentioned, in which the body is alternately showered with cold and warm water. Frequent trips to the sauna, where sweating is intentionally induced for the purpose of physiological toughening, may also have a stabilizing effect. In cases of thermoregulatory hyperhidrosis, regular sauna baths have a demonstrably therapy-enhancing effect.

There are many other traditional healing methods which also improve the chances of recovery. It is undisputed that these household remedies can contribute within certain limits to alleviating hyperhidrosis. Nevertheless, it should not be forgotten that pathological perspiration is a serious disease requiring therapy, whose treatment belongs in the hands of professional and experienced therapists.

2.6 Controlling stress

The importance of stress and emotional burdens in cases of hyperhidrosis has already been discussed in the first part of this book. In this context, the autonomic nervous systems was specified as the control unit of sweat secretion. Overcoming stress by special exercises as concurrent therapeutic measures therefore has great significance.

In connection with the psychosomatic structure of hyperhidrosis, it has already been pointed out that emotional factors that are experienced by the subjects with individually differing stress quality and quantity may be (co)responsible for a disturbance of the sweat gland function. This suggests the inverse conclusion that emotionally and mentally strengthening factors may have a healing effect.

Many forms of relaxation therapy are aimed precisely at this effect. The human psyche is capable of influencing the body, because physical relaxation and rest often have emotional relaxation and stability as a result. Since the interrelations and psychosomatic laws amplified in the first part of this book can also be extrapolated to the clinical picture of hyperhidrosis, relaxation procedures are indicated as concurrent therapy.

Relaxation therapies demonstrably have a therapeutic supportive function, but usually they do not suffice as exclusive therapy for hyperhidrosis. Their great advantage is the simplicity of execution and the fact that the unpleasant side effects frequently occurring during treatment with drugs are excluded.

There are large number of relaxation therapies, whose effect, however, is always based on the interplay between psyche and physis.

The best known relaxation techniques include bioenergetics, progressive muscular relaxation, yoga or autogenic training. The latter is presented in the following as an example for the other relaxation techniques.

Autogenic training

Autogenic training (AG) is one of the best-known relaxation techniques for achieving physical well-being at low cost. The training counteracts stress and anxieties with high effectiveness. Since fear and stress are the primary causal factors of excessive perspiration, hyperhidrotics should familiarize themselves with this relaxation technique.

AG is used primarily for prophylactic purposes. With a fast "Switch-off at will" one succeeds to some degree in countering the demands and challenges of everyday life and the professional world. After a successful learning process one can cause a mental switch-off and an escape from everyday stresses even under the most difficult conditions, which has a beneficial effect, especially in the case of the more frequently encountered clinical picture of emotional hyperhidrosis.

Stress and anxiety are frequently the cause of nervous irritability. The annoying symptom of sweat secretion is often the result precisely of emotional and physical tensions and states of stress. The excessive perspiration impressively reflects a state of tension in which the human organism finds itself in a state of alarm or even panic. AG here has the function of relaxing the muscles and calming the mind and may be understood as the reverse or transformation process for achieving a state of equilibrium.

Correct practicing of the relaxation technique removes the sounding board for stressful situations. The performance of muscle relaxation achieves an antagonistic effect. By the consciously and intentionally induced relaxation the human body passes during the exercise into an increasingly deeper state of rest, which can be further intensified with increasing practice.

The actual goal of AG is to transfer this calmness and equilibrium gradually to everyday life, thus allowing the person to achieve greater relaxation.

To illustrate the relaxing effect, it is necessary to explain a principle of psychobiology. It states that all thoughts, emotions and conceptions have the tendency to realize themselves at the physical level.

This psychobiological principle may also be regarded as interplay between action and reaction, between cause and effect. The cause is the thought, while the effect is the physical or mental reaction to this thought. The reactions may even be manifested in the organ system of the person.

In AG, the skeletal muscles and the body vessels are selectively relaxed by the power of imagination, whereby numerous variants of this anti-stress training exist today.

Most of the failures in dealing with AG are based on an unsystematic application. It is necessary to practice persistently, goal-directed, and systematically. Only then can a symptom-reducing and therefore life-enriching success be attained.

For instance, one can practice systematically by monitoring the training according to a timetable, recording the results of practice in a protocol, and thereby consciously come to terms with AG.

3.   Psychotherapy for hyperhidrosis

In psychological counseling and treatment practice, the tendency toward outbreaks of excessive perspiration is a frequently discussed physical symptom, although it is frequently discussed in connection with other symptoms and more rarely described as an exclusive and isolated phenomenon by the person seeking therapy.

The emotional life of the person is a profoundly complex and relatively unresearched area, about which multi-faceted theories exist. The consensus of the different interpretations is that disruption and overloading of the emotional life may be the cause of pathological symptoms.

The human mind is very difficult to define conceptually but can quite generally be conceived of as a superordinate sphere of human existence that influences all levels of being. Its dynamic effects are extremely complicated. They pervade all levels of human life and influence each other, so that the genesis of a disease can be explained as a consequence of mental derailments.

An emotional hyperhidrotic reacts expressively to his individual problem situation with excessive sweat secretion, which may be understood as a consequence of excessive mental pressure and as an indicator of an inner discrepanies.

The causes leading to the excessive mental demands are very diverse and may be paralleled by discrepancies in terms of basic human needs, such as respect, love, success and sexuality, and also by stress in occupational, familial and social life. The foundations of conflicts are usually laid during childhood and adolescence, which has already been mentioned concerning neurosis theory in the first part of this book.

Since mental/psychological factors can influence hyperhidrosis, an exclusively medical and symptom-oriented treatment of the disorder is not always sufficient. Therefore, besides medical analysis of the pathological sweating, a psychological examination and – if necessary – treatment of the subject should be effected simultaneously.

The psychological sequela of hyperhidrosis such as depression and other mood disorders also clearly demonstrate the necessity for a differential diagnostic approach. However, the reverse is also true. If organic causes of hyperhidrosis can be assumed during psychological therapy, a physical examination should be performed.

Psychotherapy deals exclusively with the mental and psychosomatic causes of human suffering and, in doing so, utilizes mental means of administration. These mental means include, besides the psychotherapeutic discussion – psychotherapy is frequently also called verbal medicine – all other communication processes such as nonverbal or scenic information. In psychotherapy, psychopharmaceuticals are frequently administered for the treatment of hyperhidrosis. This must basically be done under constant medical supervision.

In psychotherapy, a sort of working alliance between the treatment provider, the psychotherapist, and the patient is established, the organization of which plays a supporting role in the success of the treatment. The psychotherapeutic relationship is the foundation for achieving the therapeutic goal, because, without a one-to-one trust, sincerity and humaneness in the therapy alliance, a reduction of suffering or even relief of symptoms can hardly be accomplished.

For this reason, the demands on the professional competence of the psychotherapist, his training and experience, are high.

Even in everyday life a discussion of problems with friends or in the family circle is beneficial and unburdening, emotionally liberating. This function is precisely the focal point of psychotherapy, albeit under necessary expert guidance, because the complex emotional life of a person can only be analyzed by competent procedure. Lack of experience and a layman's attitude may do great harm here.

The primary goal of psychotherapy is to enable the patients to gain insight into their own emotional life, to provide interpretations and clarifications, to make the patients aware of their conflicts, which is the chief causes of their suffering. These subliminal conflicts buried in the subconscious become apparent to the patient, and thus the psychological pressure underlying the suffering, which until then expressed itself through the function of the sweat glands, can be substantially relieved. In the ideal case, the patients have an "aha experience," whereby the mysterious phenomena of their suffering suddenly become more clearly explainable.

The methodology of psychotherapy is therefore also frequently understood as a technique for uncovering concealed emotional contents.

The patients are given emotional support by means of psychotherapy; they gain insight into their individual emotional life, their behavior and their worldview. Psychotherapy is therefore also a constructive living tool of high prophylactic worth.

The psychotherapeutic exchange between therapist and patient takes place within the framework of procedural sessions. At regular intervals the patient meets with the psychotherapist, at which time the latter will make an effort to discover the relationships between the emotional life and the organ language expressed by the disease.

An elementary requirement imposed on the patients within the framework of the psychotherapy sessions is that they not merely be passive. Rather, they are supposed to contribute actively to the success of the psychotherapy, because only by means of the personal, honest contribution of the patient is a satisfactory therapeutic result possible.

Another requirement of patients undergoing psychotherapy is the disclosure of all events in their lives that are relevant for the pathological process, even if some of the subjects may involve pain and embarrassment, and discussing them requires overcoming a high inhibition threshold. However, such subjects are precisely elementary for psychotherapy. They permit approaches to the analysis that are highly promising of success and thus may contribute substantially to relieving the situation of suffering.

These basic rules originate from psychology and the theory of psychoanalysis, but also extend to most other directions or trends in psychotherapy. There are many psychotherapeutic procedures that will not be mentioned here since we are concerned only with the function of psychotherapy and its relevance within the scope of the treatment of hyperhidrosis.

No generalization can be made as to which psychotherapy process will come under consideration for a hyperhidrotic. Here, the individual case is the key; moreover, cost factors (not all therapy procedures are covered by health insurance) and the time frame of the treatment also play a decisive role in the choice of therapy.

Since the pressure of suffering of a hyperhidrotic is very high, several years of treatment, such as classical psychoanalysis envisions, appears unreasonably long for the situation of the afflicted. The time factor is taken into account by the process of short-term psychotherapy for the treatment of acute problems. Sometimes it includes only a few weekly sessions. A shorter treatment time also does not have be less effective than long-term therapy.

Psychotherapy is a healing process which, alone or in combination with other therapies, may contribute effectively to alleviating hyperhidrosis and especially emotional hyperhidrosis.

4. Diagnostics and objective measurement procedures

Besides a medical examination with the goal of differentiating between a case of primary or secondary hyperhidrosis, a complete case history is necessary for the diagnosis of hyperhidrosis. As mentioned above, the diagnosis of hyperhidrosis depends considerably on the subjective perception of the afflicted. Many medical practitioners collect these subjective data in the form of anamnesis forms, which the patient fills out in the waiting room.

Besides the case history, the clinical findings and the subjective statements, objective measurements also contribute to making an optimal diagnosis.

In clinical practice, the use of so-called sweat tests has become established for the purpose of quantitative and qualitative determination of the sweat quantity. These tests are an important prerequisite for the diagnosis and classification of a perspiration disorder and allow an objective evaluation of the disease. Such control procedures are also employed preoperatively for assessment of the prospects of success of an operation.

The visual orientation based on the size of the sweat spots on the clothing for the diagnosis of the axillary hyperhidrotic syndrome, is only of secondary importance, because there are many imponderable factors in play. It serves only as a rough guideline in a preliminary evaluation.

Clinical procedures for determination of the sweat quantity, besides serving diagnostic purposes, also permit the verification of therapeutic successes. Such measurements are simple to perform and require little time. These studies may also be used in combination for optimizing diagnosis and treatment.

The most widely used methods for determining the intensity of secretion include the iodine-starch test according to Minor, the copy paper method, and the gravimetric measurement process with filter paper.

In the process according to Minor, first the perspiration tendency and thus the intensity of the hyperhidrosis is objectively determined by the test procedure (also called the Minor sweat test.) The goal here is to make the physiological perspiration centers visible before botulinum toxin injection or other surgical procedure such as removal of the sweat gland zone.

In this procedure, an iodine/potassium iodide solution is applied to the skin and dusted with starch powder after drying. In the areas where the sweat glands are highly concentrated, the solution mixes with the starch. This chemical process causes a stain that makes the sweat centers with the highest gland density visible.

This test allows the determination of the extent of the hyperhidrotic zone. The difference in color between the sweat zones and the surrounding dry skin regions is quite impressive. The area can then be circled with a waterproof marker. The subsequent surgery or Botox injection can then be administered selectively. The Minor test is preferentially employed in the case of axillary hyperhidrosis. Besides this, however, the hands, feet, and even larger skin areas can be subjected to such a test.

The secretion concentration can also be distinctively documented with prepared (impregnated) plain copy paper. Flat skin regions, such as hands and feet, are especially suited for this process, in which prints are made on iodine-treated paper.

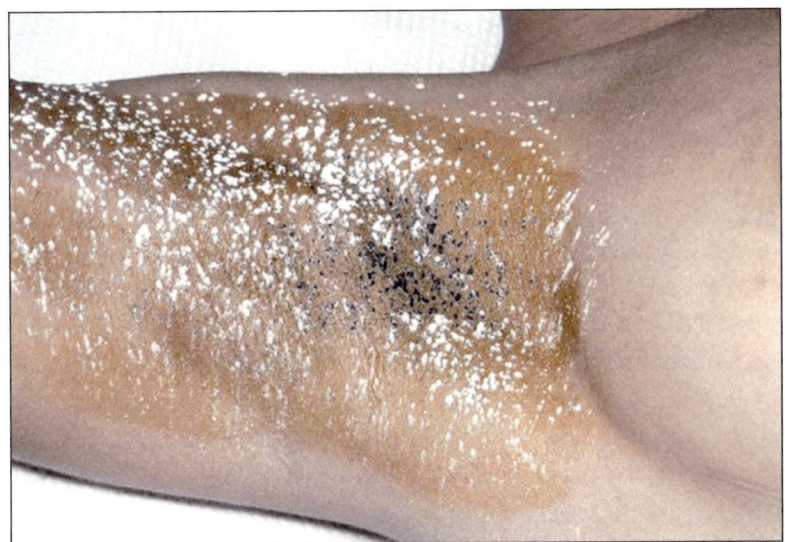

Fig. 6   Axillary iodine-starch test (Minor's sweat test.)

An alternative form of determining the sweat quantity is a gravimetric process with the aid of absorptive filter paper. The quantity of sweat secreted under thermal stimulation is collected and the quantitative secretion intensity determined by the weight gain of the paper per minute. This measurement process is especially suitable for cases of circumscribed hyperhidrosis (hands, feet, armpits.)

The secretion value above which pathological hyperhidrosis may be assumed is still debated both in the literature and in medical practice. The values are frequently set very high and difficult to reach in clinical tests. If the diagnosis is limited exclusively to achieving a measured value, then the overall evaluation of the sweat disorder is not given consideration. A secretion rate of 10–20 mg/min in the armpit region may signify a pathological axillary hyperhidrosis. A case of hyperhidrosis may be diagnosed at values of 30–40 mg/min on the hands and feet. The gravimetric test permits an assessment of the severity and a confirmation of focal hyperhidrosis at little cost.

A modern procedure that is applicable for almost any area of the body is the dynamic sweat volume measurement (quantitative sudometry) according to Dr. Schick, P.D. In this test, a computer registers the quantities of moisture secreted in several regions of the body where measurement points have been placed. This makes it possible, on the one hand, to describe the perspiration as a dynamic process in the course of time, and on the other hand, in this way, a "sweat pattern" can be set up as an individual profile. This measurement method permits one to distinguish a regional hyperhidrosis (only of the hands, for example) from a whole-body or generalized hyperhidrosis. Since generalized hyperhidrosis is a contraindication for a blockade operation of the sympathicus nerves, this test may serve as a guide for the therapy.

This costly procedure is presently offered only by the German Hyperhidrosis Center, the DHHZ, in Munich.

5. Drug-based therapies

There are scarcely any patterns of symptoms or complaints that cannot be treated pharmacologically, whether as concurrent or combined therapy. Although the pharmacology of hyperhidrosis is still a relatively new and unresearched field, various drugs have already been tested for the treatment of sweat gland disorders, most of which have a perspiration-inhibiting effect. One generally distinguishes between drugs which are homeopathic, mostly plant-derived substances, naturopathic remedies, and classic "chemical" medicine.

Medication for hyperhidrosis is usually administered by ingestion of tablets or application of ointments, emulsions, powders or creams. Drug treatment is preferred in cases of generalized hyperhidrosis, while external or topical pharmaceuticals are indicated for the treatment of localized forms. One speaks of topical therapy when, as opposed to systemic therapy, the medication is only applied or introduced locally. Topical treatment usually results in fewer side effects than systemic therapy, because a high concentration of the active principle is only achieved in a circumscribed area of the body.

5.1 Local therapy of hyperhidrosis

Perspiration-reducing preparations are known in technical medical terms as antihidrotics or antiperspirants and belong predominantly to the indication group of dermatics. Their therapeutic efficacy depends on individual factors and tolerances, and therefore their healing effect is limited.

Astringents belong to the class of locally active antihidrotics. These are the tannins, which have a constricting (astringent) effect that not only inhibits inflammation but also reduces sweat secretion.

Natural tannins are present in large amounts in the leaves and bark of oak and willow trees. Tannin contents are also present in the sage plant. The astringent effect of the tannins leads to the sealing of the sweat gland pore and thereby to the reduction of sweat formation.

The tannins precipitate or bind proteins from organic materials, so that the skin is coated with a leatherlike membrane. It is literally tanned. A compact boundary layer is created which forms an artificial horny layer (stratum corneum.)

Tannins are used primarily externally for the treatment of excessive perspiration – both in local and in whole-body treatment. From the therapeutic point of view, baths with extracts of tannin-containing plants are especially recommended for supportive treatment of generalized hyperhidrosis.

Besides plant substances, there are also a large number of synthetic tannins that are available in the form of liquid or powdered ready-to-use medications. The best-known preparations that are indicated for hyperhidrosis are listed in the appendix of this book.

Aluminum chloride and other metal compounds (zinc, magnesium) are among the most successful antiperspirants in the local therapy of hyperhidroses. They should be the drug of choice in the therapy plan, especially in cases of hyperhidrosis axillaris, manuum, and pedum. They are sold as ready-to-use products in various combinations or as an individual formulation.

The compound aluminum chloride hexahydrate ($AlCl_3$) has a very effective antihidrotic action and must be distinguished from the less effective aluminum hydroxychloride. The latter is used predominantly in the field of cosmetics. The metal salts are frequently confused.

Metal compounds have an astringent effect. They prevent and impede the discharge of secretions and may also be administered in a treatment-friendly manner in various application forms. As opposed to the systemic drugs, such as the anticholinergic or psychopharmaceuticals discussed in the following, metal compounds do not intervene in the physiological functioning of the sweat glands. They are used exclusively externally for topical application.

Application of aluminum chloride hexahydrate causes the formation of metal-mucopolysaccharide complexes in the outer skin, which fill the efferent ducts of the sweat glands as precipitate. A conglomerate of this precipitate and the degenerated epithelial cells near the walls forms a firmly adhering plug. Metal ions of the solution penetrate into the efferent ducts of eccrine sweat glands and after reaction there forms a precipitate. Protein is precipitated there, which functionally seals off the efferent ducts of the glands in the upper/outer region of the skin. Total closing of the glands due to protein decomposition is not achieved and is also not therapeutically desirable, since the biological function of perspiration should not be totally suppressed. Total sealing of the glands could lead to dangerous hyperthermia.

Another effect of the application of metal compounds, besides the mechanical closing of the efferent ducts, is the regression of secretor cells of the sweat glands.

The substances have only a superficial effect on the skin and are totally unobjectionable toxicologically and systemically.

After repeated application of metal compounds in many patients the previously high sweat flow in the affected regions of the skin is reduced.

A major drawback to the use of metal compounds, however, is the necessity of constant repetition of the application in order to maintain the result of the treatment. An achieved blocking and partial closing of the sweat gland ducts soon reverts due to the regenerative processes of the skin, so that the sweat gland excretion organs are exposed again. The original secretion can then re-establish itself. Therefore, a high measure of discipline and patience must be exercised during the treatment.

Metal compounds are sold in a variety of application forms: as solutions, creams, lotions or powders. They are available in an alcohol or aqueous solution as solvents. The aqueous solution has been proven to have the fewest side effects and is therefore the preferred solution form.

Aluminum chloride solutions for external treatment of hyperhidrosis may be used not only in the liquid state but also as a viscous gel. In gel form, this substance can even be packaged in a deodorant roll-on stick, which greatly simplifies application to the skin. As a rule the metal solution is prepared by a pharmacist and often enriched with additional substances. Due to the variety of application forms of aluminum chloride hexahydrate, the latter may be adapted to the specific local perspiration symptoms of the subject.

Various formulations for these solutions may be found in the pharmaceutical literature. In some countries, there are scientifically tested formulation guidelines that are subject to constant revision. Doctors and pharmacists are sufficiently familiar with these guidelines, so that the subject should not be motivated in any way to prepare the solution himself. The following standardized formulations exist in Germany on the basis of the NRF (Neues Rezeptur-Formularium,) whose composition is known to all German pharmacists.

- Aluminum chloride hexahydrate gel 15 % / 20 %, NRF 11.24
- 2-propanol-containing aluminum chloride hexahydrate solution 15 % / 20 %, NRF 11.1
- Viscous aluminum chloride hexahydrate solution 15 % / 20 %, NRF 11.132

The gel and the viscous solution are alcohol-free. The basis of the alcohol solution contains 80% 2-propanol (V/V). However, lower-alcohol and alcohol-free aqueous solutions can certainly also be produced.

In many individual formulations, the admixture of silicone oil is recommended for reducing the sensitization rate. This additive is possible only in alcohol-based preparations; it cannot be incorporated in purely aqueous preparations. Although silicone oil is present in many skin care products, and this may be related to an improvement in skin tolerance, this is detrimental to the effect of aluminum chloride. For this reason, such additives are intentionally omitted in the NRF. If, contrary to expectations, intolerance/ incompatibility should occur, it is advisable first to lower the concentration. In the case of very sensitive skin, the concentration may be reduced down to 3%.

Hydroxyethylcellulose (HEC) and not methylcellulose, as often described in the literature, is used exclusively for gel production and for viscosity modification. If a change in viscosity is desired, the concentration of the HEC is adjusted accordingly. This is accomplished, for instance, with the two NRF formulations 11.24 (solid gel) and 11.132 (viscous solution.)

If axillary hyperhidrosis is present, a roll-on applicator containing the metal mixture or a pad dispenser is the ideal form of application. Hyperhidrosis of the hands and/or feet, as opposed to this, would be better treated by using a liquid metal solution, since the liquid can manifest its sweat-inhibiting effect on these skin regions much more intensively and can penetrate more deeply into the skin surface, and thereby into the gland secretor organs. If patients have questions as to the optimal dosage and the right application form of the metal-based active principles, they can turn to either doctors or pharmacists.

Administration of a solution containing aluminum chloride hexahydrate is the treatment of choice in therapeutic practice and, above all, in the individual treatment of excessive sweat secretion, and is indicated for axillary and palmo-plantar hyperhidrosis, best results being achieved in the case of the former. In dermatological test series, a significant reduction in sweat secretion was achieved in approximately 90% of the patients suffering from hyperhidrosis axillaris by application of metal salts.

Depending on intensity and localization of the hyperhidrosis, a solution with aluminum chloride hexahydrate can be administered in different concentrations. The healing effect is directly proportional to the content of aluminum chloride in this case. The decisive factor is the tolerance for the agent. If skin irritation occurs, the concentration or the solvent may be changed. In the case of milder symptoms of sweat gland hyperfunction, the concentration of 10–15% $AlCl_3$ is sufficient to reduce the secretion rate. Intensive hyperhidrosis cases, on the other hand, should be treated with a higher concentration, up to a maximum 30%, the highest concentration being considered for application to hands and feet. A formulation with aluminum chloride has a strong acid and antiseptic effect. In the alcohol solution, the substance does not decompose as readily as in aqueous ones, although the application of moisturizing creams is frequently necessary due to the drying-out effect of the alcohol solution. If the skin does not tolerate the astringent, it should be attempted to switch to an aqueous solution or to reduce the alcohol concentration.

Aluminum chloride solution is exclusively for external application and should be applied to the affected skin areas just before going to bed. At this time the sweat glands are predominantly dormant, which is especially true in the case of emotional hyperhidrosis. In this resting phase, the metal substance can diffuse optimally into the sweat gland excretory ducts, where it manifests its antihidrotic effect. Immediate flushing out or sweating out of the solution is avoided. The residues can be washed off in the morning.

When administered in viscous form, the metal compound is massaged into the skin areas. Roughly one fingertip of gel is often sufficient and should not be rubbed in for longer than 30 seconds. In the liquid state, the solution can also be applied by hand and massaged in the same way. Swabbing the solution on with a cotton pad is recommended for sensitive areas of the skin.

This application should initially be performed every 2–3 days or daily in the case of very persistent hyperhidrosis. The time interval of application should be several months, so that the substance can develop its full effect.

The aluminum chloride solution has a pleasant extra function. An antibacterial effect produced by the solution suppresses unpleasant sweat odor. The antiperspirant is therefore also indicated in cases of bromhidrosis.

On the whole, the application of metal salts is a suitable and effective means for controlling excessive perspiration. The treatment can be self-administered and, for this reason, is also accepted in the inner circle of therapeutic measures. The cost is low and the application also has scarcely any side effects, so that the harm-benefit ratio is optimal.

In isolated cases, skin erythema, itching and blistering may occur. Usually, these reactions subside when the concentration is reduced.

Aluminum chloride in a high-percentage alcohol solution has a greater tendency to cause sensitization disorders than in aqueous solution. On the other hand, the substances decompose more slowly in water, and skin-irritating acids may form.

Metal salts may also cause edema or mild inflammations. Such symptoms are experienced as an itching sweat rash caused by the plugging of the sweat gland ducts. Blisters may form due to sweat congestion, which burst and dry up relatively quickly. Such side effects, however, are the exception. They may be countered when necessary with creams and skin-protective lotions. Patients mistakenly believe they are still sweating, although objectively a non-pathological state (normhidrosis) already exists.

Another side effect is that metal solutions are corrosive and can cause discoloration/stains on textiles, especially when used on the armpits. However, this drawback can be avoided by proper and careful application of the solution.

Formaldehyde and formalin have a similar antihidrotic effect to that of aluminum chloride, but they are less frequently used because of allergic contact reactions on the skin surface.

Besides the individual formulations, many commercial preparations exist worldwide that are based on metal compounds. For the most part, these involve over-the-counter products and only in rare cases preparations requiring a prescription. The most common and most in-demand antiperspirants found in the online pharmacy are listed in the appendix of this book.

5.2 Plant-derived therapeutic agents

Homeopathy as a natural healing process is an alternative treatment method, which may also be applied, in individual cases, as a concurrent therapy for hyperhidrosis.

The special characteristic of these purely herbal medicines of low risk for the patient is the fact that highly potent natural active principles are administered, which, in small doses, unfold in healthy persons precisely those symptoms that are to be controlled. As irritants, these preparations stimulate a defensive reaction in the human organism, which presupposes an intact function of the body's immune system.

Sage (Salvia officinalis,) as an herbal therapeutic agent, has been proven effective in the treatment of hyperhidrosis. One of the traditional indications for sage is sweat outbursts in adolescence. The antiperspirant effect of the sage plant is traceable in part to tannins; it also contains germicidal substances and essential oils. Sage acts on the endocrine glands as well as on the sympathic nervous system in a tranquilizing and balancing manner.

This natural remedy can be administered to the patient in many forms, as tablets or pills, as a tea, salve, oil, or drops. The antihidrotic effect of sage and other plant extracts, however, has to date not been objectivized.

The healing effect of the sage plant was already known in medieval times. Its application is very simple and pleasant, because the active principle is relatively neutral in taste and can be administered in high doses. The sweat-inhibiting effect of this plant extract is said to appear after a short time. The best-known sage preparation for the indication hyperhidrosis is Sweatosan® in the form of tablets.

The advantage of herbal medicines is that they have few side effects. The only contraindication for sage is nursing/breastfeeding mothers, since the herbal principles may stop milk production.

Herbal antihidrotics are often sold in the form of so-called sweat drops with different active principles. Even in the case of self-medication, health risks from the taking of such preparations exist only in rare cases.

Unfortunately, the therapeutic results only rarely meet the expectations of the patients. A reduction of sweat secretion can indeed be demonstrated in individual cases, but cannot be generalized. Therapeutic success is almost totally absent in the case of extreme hyperhidrosis. Milder forms of hyperhidrosis, however, may also be treated with herbal medicines.

5.3 Systemic Therapy

The chemical substances for treatment of hyperhidrosis that require a prescription include the pharmacological group of anticholinergics. Their secretion-inhibiting potential is based on the interplay of sweat glands and cholinergic nerves. The active principles of the anticholinergic substances, also called cholinergic blockers, inhibit the function of sympathic nerve fibers governing the activity of the eccrine glands by blocking the receptors on the secretor cells of the sweat glands.

Upon stimulation of the hypothalamus, the messenger substance acetylcholine is liberated at the ends of the cholinergic fibers, which is important for sweat secretion. Acetylcholine has the function of binding to the secretor cells and activating secretion by the sweat glands via complicated biochemical processes. This transmitter is presumably also responsible for activation of the electrolytes, which perform an important function in the perspiration cycle and stimulate secretion by the sweat glands.

By occupying the receptors in the sympathic ganglia with anticholinergic substances, this reaction is suppressed, so that the extent of the secretion is reduced. The excess transmitter substance is ultimately decomposed by the enzyme cholinesterase into its constituents choline and acetic acid and thereby deactivated.

The best-known active principles among the anticholinergics include bornaprine hydrochloride, atropine, scopolamine, banthine, and propantheline bromide.

Anticholinergic substances are not uniformly effective in their sweat-inhibiting action. They are indeed able to reduce sweat secretion but often not to the degree expected by the patient.

If one considers, besides the fact that anticholinergics cannot guarantee complete and long-lasting improvement, the risk of possible adverse side effects, then an anticholinergic treatment as the exclusive therapeutic measure for hyperhidrosis should only be applied after careful weighing of the advantages and disadvantages.

There is only rarely an indication for exclusive treatment with anticholinergics. These agents are administered in cases of tremor dominance (trembling) and within the framework of combination therapies. There is also an extensive list of contraindications for these substances.

Anticholinergics are not therapeutically selective in their effect; therefore, they are not only sweat gland secretion inhibitors. The also act on a large number of action sites and, therefore, are used for quite different indications. The desired effect in one indication may thus lead to an adverse side effect in another.

The most common adverse side effects include:

- Accommodation problems (vision disturbances)
- Unpleasant xerostomia (dry mouth)
- Allergic skin reactions
- Negative psychotropic effects
- Tachycardia (heart racing)
- Constipation (retained stool)
- Bladder evacuation problems

In therapeutic practice, anticholinergics are used in cases of strong generalized hyperhidrosis. However, for hyperhidrosis of other genesis and location, the use of an anticholinergic drug may also produce entirely satisfactory results, as has been demonstrated in a large number of clinical studies of the therapeutic effect of bornaprine. Compared to other anticholinergics, the drug bornaprine has the fewest side effects. Bornaprine has a very pronounced anticholinergic efficacy which has been tested in the treatment of Parkinsonism and in hyperhidrosis as a sequela of spinal-lesion paraplegia. A drug widely used in Europe that contains this active substance is Sormodren® (among others, it is licensed in Austria, Mexico, Spain, Ireland, Italy, and Germany.) This is an anticholinergic that is frequently prescribed for generalized hyperhidrosis without organic findings. Good results can be achieved if it is administered in carefully measured doses under medical supervision.

The dosage has direct consequences not only for tolerance but also for the time of onset of the effect. By rapidly increasing the dose, an earlier onset of the effect can be achieved, which, however, is accompanied by more autonomic disorders, which may sometimes be extremely unpleasant. Therefore, when selecting the form of medication, good tolerance for the preparation should be given priority over the fast therapeutic effect desired by the patient.

Excessive perspiration is listed among the indications for this drug today, but originally it was a drug for the treatment of the tremor in Parkinson's disease (elevated muscle tone, palsy.) The preparation should therefore only be prescribed with corresponding information about the numerous possible side effects.

Besides bornaprine, the anticholinergic agent methanthelinum bromide (Vagantin®) is also one of the better known drugs in the therapy for excessive perspiration.

The drugs prescribed for hyperhidrosis also include the atropine derivatives, although hyperhidrosis is not listed as an indication in their user information. Atropine is used primarily for internal diseases and in ophthalmology. Atropine is an alkaloid that occurs in many plants of the nightshade variety. Drugs with this ingredient are occasionally used therapeutically in hyperhidrosis because of their possible secondary effect of sweat inhibition. Atropine paralyzes the acetylcholine receptors in the synapses, has a spasmolytic effect, and thereby also curbs secretion processes.

In view of the possible side effects of this drug, e.g., dry mouth, heat buildup, vision problems, skin erythema, heart palpitation, and psychological disturbances such as agitation and hallucinations, every doctor should inform his/her patient about alternative means or methods of treatment.

Atropine as an active principle is also not specific in its sweat-reducing effect. In general, it acts as a cholinergic blocker and, therefore, not only causes a reduction in function of the sweat glands but also impairs other glands.

Glycopyrrolate, or its active principle glycopyrronium bromide (Robinul®) is another anticholinergic that may be used in hyperhidrosis. In scientific studies, the efficacy of local application of glycopyrrolate in the form of a solution or cream was investigated in connection with the Frey syndrome.

This drug is occasionally used to reduce the flow of saliva before initiation of anesthesia. The active principle has a drying effect, not only on the oral mucosa but also on the skin of the entire body and may be taken orally (Robinul forte®) to relieve sweating. The side effects are comparable with those of the aforementioned anticholinergics. Application should be avoided in the case of a high outdoor temperature, since thermoregulatory perspiration may be noticeably impaired.

Propantheline bromide (Pro-Banthine®) also belongs to the group of anticholinergics with the effect of pharmacological inhibition of the functions of the sympathic nervous system and, therefore, also of reducing hyperhidrosis. The preparation is occasionally used for treatment of hypertension.

The drug clonidine from the group of antihypertensives also belongs to the nonspecific drugs used in systemic therapy. This is a drug used to treat high blood pressure and relieve withdrawal symptoms in drug or alcohol withdrawal therapy. The drug causes the blood vessels to dilate, reduces the heart rate, and lowers blood pressure. Clonidine (Catapresan®) can be administered orally or intravenously. The pharmacological effects of this substance include, among others, the lowering of the sympathicotonia by reduced secretion of norepinephrine.

A systemic therapy with the drugs named above will not be disputed or advised against here, despite the nonspecific mode of action and the possible, sometimes serious, side effects; the pressure of the suffering of the afflicted is too great and the simplicity of such medication too seductive.

Nevertheless, caution is urged when taking such drugs and then only under the strictest medical supervision. The sudden discontinuation of drugs containing these substances may also provoke serious disorders.

For a doctor, such "pill therapy" is advantageous from the economic and organizational standpoint, because prescribing is simple. Often general practitioners hastily give such drugs to their patients who present the history of their complaint during consultation, although alternative effective treatments are an option in many forms of hyperhidrosis. Here, the patient is also urged not to rashly demand such a drug treatment.

The high pressure due to the suffering with which the hyperhidrotic is afflicted is often the cause of the treatment with anticholinergics, atropine derivatives, or antihypertensives. If the afflicted is given the prospect of help by the apparently simple taking a pill, then, after visiting the doctor, often a dangerous experimental procedure is carried out. In self-medication, the dosage is varied, because the patients now believe they can finally rid themselves of their burden of suffering. Uncontrolled medication with this highly potent substance, however, entails the great risk of physical harm. This problem has increased against the background of easy access to even prescription-requiring medications via the Internet. The subjects are thus exposed to a great temptation that may have far-reaching consequences for their health.

5.4 Psychopharmaceuticals

Psychopharmaceuticals are the most frequently prescribed drugs, although they entail a high risk potential for the patients. These drugs are also frequently prescribed when hyperhidrosis is present.

It is undeniable that emotional perspiration can be effectively treated with centrally sedative, therefore tranquilizing and anxiety-relieving drugs. The best-known psychopharmaceuticals with a tranquilizing and excitation-reducing action are the tranquilizers, antidepressives, and neuroleptics. Such drugs should be administered, if at all, only by competent practitioners or psychotherapists familiar with the application.

Psychopharmaceuticals have a psychotropic effect, since they intervene in the human brain metabolism. Their active principles influence differentiated biochemical processes that are controlled by the central nervous system.

The phenomenon of excessive perspiration therefore does not belong to the strict indication of psychopharmaceuticals. A reduction of the sweat secretion is rather achieved secondarily from the taking of these drugs.

Psychopharmaceuticals in the initial phase of therapy cause a spontaneous reduction or even elimination of symptoms. At little cost the prescribing doctor can restore the desired functional fitness of the patient in a relatively short time.

However, this state, which is perceived as "liberating," usually does not last. Often the symptoms concealed by the psychopharmaceuticals reappear. Despite taking drugs, the hyperhidrotics then react in the emotionally stressful or fear-loaded situations typical for them with further outbreaks of sweating and, in many cases, even more intensive than before.

If the symptoms recur while still in the treatment phase, the drug dose is often increased in order to maintain the effect. Constantly increasing quantities are needed in order to maintain the previously achieved effect of perspiration inhibition. Here, a vicious circle is created that is typical for the use of many psychotherapeutically active substances.

Psychopharmaceuticals function basically as an emotional "crutch." They mask and conceal only the symptoms of hyperhidrosis, but change nothing as regards the cause of the emotional or psychogenous hyperhidrosis.

Their serious side effects testify against medication with psychopharmaceuticals. These drugs may, in the worst case, lead to addiction, with all of its concomitant symptoms. The patient then remains emotionally as well as physically dependent on these drugs. When they are discontinued, the body reacts with significant withdrawal symptoms.

The development of dependence due to inexpert administration or taking of drugs is especially quite frequent in the case of tranquilizers, which are primarily intended to relieve states of anxiety.

It should not be disputed that psychopharmaceuticals may play an important role in the treatment of hyperhidrosis. Within the framework of psychotherapy, where constant supervision is given, they may be used quite beneficially.

In this context, one should not disregard the occasionally uncritical prescription habits of doctors who use psychopharmaceuticals as long-term medication. Psychopharmaceuticals are to be used only in extremely rare cases and certainly not as long-term medication for the treatment of hyperhidrosis.

Beta-receptor blockers (for short: beta blockers) are also prescribed for the treatment of hyperhidrosis; originally used in internal medicine, but today are to be found in almost every home medicine cabinet. Beta-receptor blockers, strictly speaking, are not classical psychopharmaceutical agents.

The best-known area of application of the beta blockers is the treatment of arterial hypertension and the prevention of heart diseases. Besides this original use, however, another indication has been generally accepted, i.e., the treatment of anxiety syndromes. Precisely in the treatment of anxiety, however, one sees a potentially abusive application of these drugs, since they are frequently used "rashly," even for "speech anxiety" and "stage fright."

Beta blockers regulate and influence the emotional-mental state. They have a symptom-damping effect on the autonomic nervous system. Since the symptoms often push to the foreground in anxiety disorders, the symptom of perspiration may also be one of these autonomic anxiety symptoms.

Beta blockers have gained their current well-known status because of their spontaneous efficiency and because they, as opposed to the much-debated tranquilizers, are accompanied by only a few side effects with almost the same therapeutic effect. Simple application and immediate damping of unrest and states of agitation have contributed to the popularity of these drugs. To date no cases of addiction to beta blockers are known.

The native hormones, epinephrine and norepinephrine, are liberated at the sympathic nerve endings or from the adrenal cortex in anxiety and stress situations. The stress hormone, epinephrine, plays a decisive part in such cases. This hormone stimulates the beta receptors of the nerve cells, causing a physical state of excitation. The beta receptors are located on the cell membranes of many organs, such as the heart, vessels, kidneys, or bronchi.

If these receptors are stimulated by the transmitter substance epinephrine, then symptoms of anxiety are evoked. In the hyperhidrotic, this stimulation may be discharged by an unpleasant hypersecretion.

The active principle of the beta blockers prevents the binding of the stress hormone to the receptors, because the latter are blocked. The result is that the transmission of stimuli by epinephrine to the key points of the nerve cells is suppressed, and the symptoms of excitation are therefore relieved.

A high epinephrine concentration in the circulating blood demonstrably leads to intensified sweat secretion. Antiadrenergic substances, to which the beta blockers belong, are capable of reducing sweat secretion.

However, the trend medication with beta blockers only permits the control of visible physical symptoms. The mental factors representing the root cause of the suffering are not taken into account.

A negative concurrent physiological phenomenon is the increase in the number of receptors during long-term medication, which may result in hypersensitivity. If the medication is discontinued, the stress sensitivity may develop into so-called hypersensitivity, where even the slightest stimulus is reacted to with an extreme excitation reaction.

Reasonable control of stress is then scarcely possible, with the consequence that the tablet must be taken again, with a stronger content of active principle or in a higher dose.

Nevertheless, the beta blockers appear to be the less dangerous substances when compared with the classic psychopharmaceuticals. They may be recommended for concurrent treatment of hyperhidrosis.

In the treatment of hyperhidrosis with beta blockers, the drug propranolol (Inderal®) has been found to be especially efficacious. The beta blockers are not all equal in their effect, so that some drugs are contraindicated because they may provoke hypersecretion (symptomatic hyperhidrosis after taking medication.)

6. Physical therapy

6.1 Tap water iontophoresis

Tap water iontophoresis (TWI) is probably the most effective treatment in the spectrum of local therapies for hyperhidrosis and is among the classic conventional applications for moderate-to-high degrees of severity.

In this process, by using water baths or moist electrodes, continuous or high-frequency pulsed direct currents are passed through previously identified hyperhidrotic skin areas. The safe indications for tap water iontophoresis are primary hyperhidrosis of the palms of the hands and soles of the feet. Axillary hyperhidrosis can, with some limitations, also be effectively treated by this procedure.

In the presence of generalized hyperhidrosis this process is less advisable from the standpoint of current research. In such cases, as an alternative, hydroelectric baths are recommended as whole-body current baths. As in the case of iontophoresis, direct current at a voltage of up to 25 V is applied in this full hydroelectric bath.

The patient is in a special bathtub filled with tap water and equipped with electrodes. As opposed to iontophoresis, in which the entire current flows through the patients, in the hydroelectric bath they are only influenced by 10–30% of the current, the rest flows through the water.

Iontophoresis is a form of physical therapy whose effectiveness and therefore sweat-inhibiting effect has been scientifically thoroughly studied and confirmed. The secretion mechanism of the sweat glands is governed by electrolytes within the scope of osmotic processes between the cells of the sweat glands and their immediate surroundings.

In the course of iontophoresis treatment, ionized substances are introduced through the skin by means of electric current. At this time the flow of ions into the sweat gland excretory ducts is greatest, because the skin resistance is lowest there.

By means of this process biochemical and consequently secretion-controlling processes are unleashed, leading to inhibition of glandular secretion. The therapeutic effect is traceable to a raising of the stimulation threshold of the sweat glands. In research and science, one assumes a functional blockage of the secretor epithelium of the sweat gland.

The ion flow was accurately determined in clinical studies with the aid of dyes. Thus, it was shown that the ions are transported into the efferent ducts of the sweat glands. The exploitation of this finding is the basis of this well-known and effective form of physical therapy.

Tap water is usually used as the electric current carrier in iontophoresis. As alternatives, there are also physical procedures using other conductors. These conductive substances may be formed, e.g., with the aid of astringent medications whose active agents pass into the permeable skin due to the conduction process.

Tap water iontophoresis is preferred over other procedures, because the potential side effects are reduced to an acceptable measure in this application.

Iontophoresis therapy is used in practice as follows, here referring to hyperhidrosis of the hands and feet.

In clinical application, the patient dips hands and/or feet into a shallow plastic dish half-filled with water. Two electrodes are placed in it, which generate a weak current, causing a slight tingling sensation in the patient. By means of a current source (ionto-phoresis device,) a continuous or pulsed direct current is passed via the electrodes through the hands or feet. This current slows down the secretion by the sweat glands, whereby this sweat-reducing effect depends on the intensity of the current (usually approximately 10–15 mA) and the duration of the treatment.

Depending on the apparatus, a treatment will last about 10–30 minutes, and should initially be applied daily, or at least two to four times per week, in order to achieve a satisfactory result.

The therapeutic effect with pulsed current is somewhat less compared to continuous direct current, but it is sufficient for treatment of moderate-grade hyperhidrosis. This limitation can be compensated, depending on the apparatus, by increasing the voltage at the same dose setting adjustment, so that the therapy with pulsed current is also suitable for stronger forms of hyperhidrosis.

The local unpleasant sensations possibly felt during the treatment, such as tingling, burning or the so-called "low-voltage pasture fence" effect that may occur upon immersion or removing of the hands or feet into or out of the treatment dish due to voltages jumps do not or hardly ever occur during pulsed therapy. This is, therefore, the preferred method for children and patients whose current sensitivity is higher.

The application of this physical process should be variably configured, corresponding to the severity of the hyperhidrosis in each case and to the individual circumstances, and any changes in the application of the process should be made in consultation with the treating dermatologist.

Sweat formation will normalize already after 10–15 applications. There is, however, the disadvantage that the effect of sweat inhibition after intensive therapy subsides relatively quickly, and thus necessitates maintenance therapy. Individual differences exist as regards the time intervals of the repetitions. In practice, a repetition rate of one to two times per week has proven favorable.

Even in axillary hyperhidrosis, extraordinary improvements are achieved with iontophoresis. Current treatment under the arms, however, requires a special form of therapy, above all with respect to the equipment and the quality of the electrodes that have to be affixed in the armpits.

The therapy is more difficult in the axillary region than in cases of planoplantar hyperhidrosis, because the skin is much more sensitive here. High therapeutic currents may here cause current marks and slight reddening. Upon diagnosis of a pronounced case of axillary hyperhidrosis this application should be considered for inclusion in the therapy and at least tested for its effect.

In a few cases, circumscribed forms of hyperhidrosis even exceeding the actual indication have been treated by using special equipment. Further dermatological research results concerning the many applications of this form of physical therapy are still unavailable since the research time frames are very long. Another method involves treatment of the face and head region characterized by special applicator devices (face masks, etc.)

The advantage of iontophoresis therapy compared to other therapeutic measures is predominantly its problem-free application. Another benefit is that this procedure, as opposed to drug therapy or surgery, can be administered almost completely without side effects. The treatment is therefore risk-free and, in most cases, highly effective.

The few and rare side effects include a mild burning or stinging, blistering on the skin, and minor skin irritation. This appears quite tolerable when compared with the side effects of drug therapy or a neurosurgical operation. By using tap water iontophoresis, the excessive perspiration can be substantially improved or relieved without drugs, without side effects and without surgery within a short time. Due to these obvious advantages, this technique has become the primary therapeutic measure, especially for palmoplantar hyperhidrosis.

Side effects are unknown to both patients and therapists, even after years of long-term therapy. It is recommended that pulsed direct current be selected for the treatment of children. A general prerequisite is that the children be able to understand and obey the therapy instructions. Therefore, iontophoresis treatment before the age of 6 years is usually not advisable. The few noteworthy contraindications for iontophoresis include treatment of patients with cardiac pacemakers, metal implants, or large-area skin defects. Pregnant women should also avoid this therapy.

Iontophoresis treatment appears at first glance to be complicated and costly, especially because it must first be administered under clinical supervision. In the meanwhile, however, portable iontophoresis devices for home use have been developed, which the patients can operate themselves with relative ease after receiving the proper training.

The patient is thus given the possibility of performing self-therapy at home. The health insurance will often pay for the acquisition of the device, since the result of the treatment justifies the cost, and the latter is usually less than what medical "odysseys" with an uncertain outcome and unforeseeable costs would involve.

6.2 Hidrex®-Therapy

High technical requirements must be met when choosing therapeutic devices for conducting tap water iontophoresis in clinical practice. Depending on the manufacturer, the devices display serious differences. This pertains primarily to wear, patient safety, operator friendliness and hygienic conditions.

These features should therefore be taken into account when selecting a suitable therapy device, so that the therapeutic effect is not impeded by technical problems. Clinicians and practitioners are normally familiar with the guidelines of iontophoresis therapy and are aware of the high requirements imposed on an efficient device. The firm Hidrex GmbH of Heiligenhaus, Germany, is one of the leading manufacturers of iontophoresis devices.

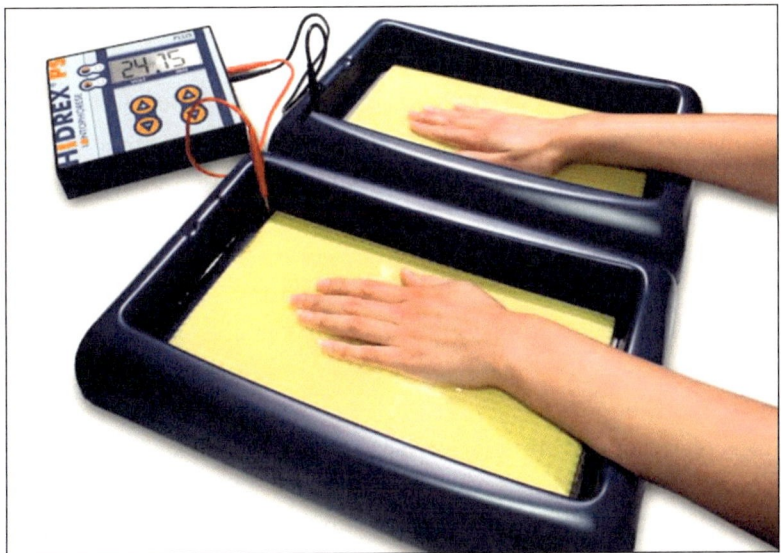

Fig. 7   Iontophoresis treatment of the hands in a special bath exemplified byHidrex® therapy.

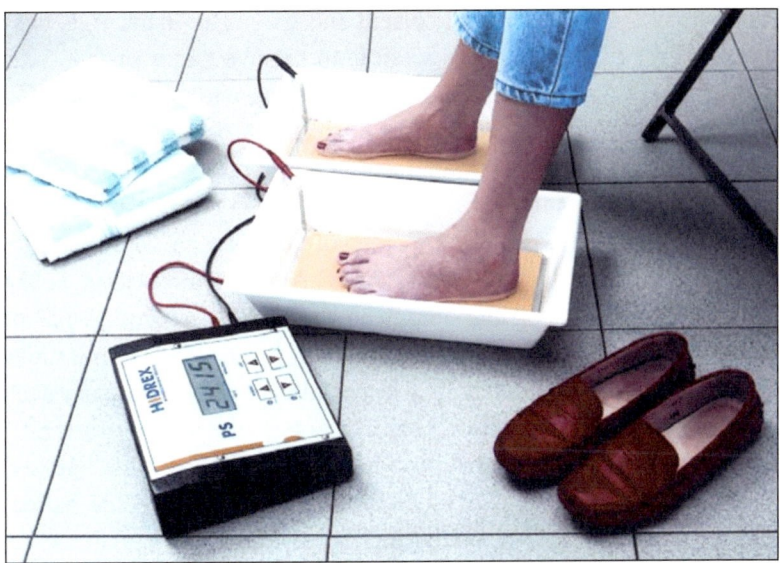

Fig. 8   Iontophoresis treatment of the feet in a special bath exemplified by Hidrex® therapy.

Hidrex® devices satisfy the high technical requirements for clinical practice and are characterized by simple operation and reliability with the highest effectiveness.

In many dermatological clinics, these devices are therefore the first choice because they are developed with application of high safety standards in cooperation with the largest university clinics of Germany. The devices made by the Hidrex Company have been found in comparative tests to be highly worthy of recommendation due to their high performance and best therapeutic efficiency.

Besides the classical direct-current devices with high flexibility, the pulsed-current (PS) Hidrex® devices, in particular, are characterized by their innovative current flow. This specific form of current was developed by the company and first used about 10 years ago. These devices emit pulses of direct current with a physiologically favorable frequency. The previously experienced sensation of actually feeling the therapeutic current is almost totally eliminated here. However, the efficacy of the application is still just as high. With both the direct-current and the pulsed-current devices of the Hidrex Company it is possible to remove hands or feet from the treatment dish while the current is flowing without experiencing the so-called "picket fence" effect. Hidrex® devices, in contrast with devices by other manufacturers, operate with a specific regulation that suppresses voltage fluctuations. The current intensity can be adapted to personal desires and is limited to maximal values to avoid safety risks. Another innovation is the possibility of reducing the output power to 50% for both types of current. Cutting the rate of current buildup in half tends to minimize its perception. The treatment of especially sensitive patients, such as children, for example, or sensitive zones of the body (armpits) can thus be performed even more individually and gently. Currently, there also exists a unique device with which the patient himself can vary the dosage during the therapy session. The newer devices include the GS Classic® and the PS Plus® models, the latter being capable of switching back and forth between direct and pulsed current, permitting a voltage of up to 60 V, and therefore being equally well applicable in cases of severe hyperhidrosis. Hidrex® devices are TÜV tested, provided with the CE symbol and licensed and medical devices according to EU Guideline 93/42/EWG and the German Medical Products Law (MPG). The characteristic safety features of the devices include immersion monitoring, excess therapy protection, current increase limitation, excess current and excess voltage monitoring. Besides the well-known hand and foot baths, special armpit applicators are also available. Ergobaths, hand towels, transport cases, and hand bath switches nowadays belong to the set of accessories that come with the devices.

The treatment process of the special Hidrex® therapy is divided into two phases. In the first phase, the treatment is performed under medical supervision and the patient learns how to carry out the treatment. As a rule, the sweat secretion normalizes after about ten treatments. The medical supervision provides the proof of success of this initial phase that is frequently required by the medical insurance provider. This is then followed by the second phase, long-term therapy, which is performed at home. Its application then depends on the severity of the condition, usually one to three times weekly.

The devices may be borrowed from the Hidrex Co. for testing purposes at no cost. A rental fee becomes due after five weeks. This is the procedure currently in use at the major clinics for the initial phase of the therapy. When the device is returned, a small lump sum is charged for used materials such as hand towels, trays, and electrodes. No extra charges are levied when the device is bought (privately or through insurance.)

7. Surgical procedures

7.1 Botulinum toxin

Botulinum toxin is well known as a very strong nerve poison. Ingestion of the poison can lead to food poisoning, botulism, which may be caused by eating spoiled canned foods or sausage products from home butchering. For years botulinum toxin has been used successfully in neurology as a licensed drug for the treatment of muscle spasms and mobility problems (dystonia).

The active principle is obtained from the bacterium *Clostridium botulinum*, which produces different types of botulinum toxin. Only botulinum toxin type A is used in the therapy of hyperhidrosis. In technical terms, the designation Botox® is more widely used, which is a registered trademark of Pharm-Allergan GmbH, which sells the drug.

From the neurophysiological standpoint the toxin, when properly used, i.e., introduced into the skin by injection, inhibits the secretion of acetylcholine. Acetylcholine is the transmitter substance which triggers sweat secretion in the neurochemical process. Botox® causes a presynaptic inhibition of the secretion of acetylcholine by the binding of the active principle to the vesicle filled with acetylcholine.

Botox® thereby blocks the cholinergic nerve fibers that lead to the sweat glands. The sweat glands of the skin region treated with Botox® are thus inactivated.

Only very recently has this bacterial poison also been used for the medium-to-long-term treatment of specific hyperhidroses. The treatment of hyperhidrosis with Botox® was licensed in Germany on August 13, 2003 after multi-center clinical studies had been performed on patients with primary axillary hyperhidrosis and approved exclusively for this indication.

In the US, the active principle was tested on July 19, 2004 by the licensing authority, the FDA, and declared to be permissible for the treatment of severe axillary hyperhidrosis. In the meanwhile, Botox® has been licensed for the indication hyperhidrosis in 33 countries according to a statement by Pharm-Allergan GmbH.

The field of application of Botox® therefore includes a strong, persistent primary hyperhidrosis axillaris, which may have disturbing effects on the activities of daily life and cannot be treated adequately by topical therapy.

An absolute prerequisite for the prescription and application of this drug is that a detailed history be recorded and a physical examination performed, together with other necessary specific examinations for excluding secondary hyperhidrosis. Thus, a purely symptomatic treatment of the hyperhidrosis without diagnosis and/or without treatment of the underlying disease is avoided.

Botox® therapy is one of the more recent therapy options. This form of therapy is not yet officially permitted for more extensive indications of hyperhidrosis. The authorization of Botox® as an alternative treatment to surgery, in addition to the narrow indication of axillary hyperhidrosis, is still awaited.

Health insurance institutions/companies usually do not approve the high cost of this treatment in absence of the specific indication. In such cases, Botox® is used as a licensed medication, albeit for an indication for which it is not permitted.

Nevertheless, doctors may exercise therapeutic freedom to use a drug notwithstanding the indication if this appears medically advisable. This rule was recently upheld by large-scale studies at various dermatological clinics. A large number of patients with hyperhidrosis were treated with the bacterial toxin; the results were convincing in terms of the effectiveness of the injection therapy.

Botox® was administered in the form of injections in local hyperhidrosis. The drug is sold as a powder for preparation of the injection solution. Botox® therapy is presently a genuine alternative to surgery for relieving excessive perspiration of the hands, feet or armpits and is convincing due to its high efficacy even in the case of pronounced symptoms. The drug promises very good results in the treatment of excessive armpit sweating. Botox® injection is also used for the effective reduction of gustatory sweating.

Botox® may only be administered by doctors with the proper qualifications, demonstrated technical skills, and treatment experience. The required technical equipment must also be available. An extremely high degree of precision is required for dosing the injections and in the course of the treatment. Therefore, this injection process should only be carried out in special clinics.

Before the injection therapy itself, first, using the above-described iodine-starch test, the sweating tendency, i.e., the intensity of the hyperhidrosis, and the sweat centers (usually the armpits) must be objectively determined.

If an indication for Botox® therapy is given for the subject after having performed the sweat quantity test, depending on the local intensity of the sweat flow, the active principle is injected into the affected skin areas. Injections are made in several places of the area affected by hyperhidrosis in order to achieve the most efficient denervation possible of the sweat glands.

In most cases, local anesthesia is administered, since the injections may be painful. The result of the treatment appears only about five to six days after the injection. Unfortunately, the effect of this treatment is only temporary; studies indicate four to six months, one year at a maximum. After this time interval the procedure has to be repeated.

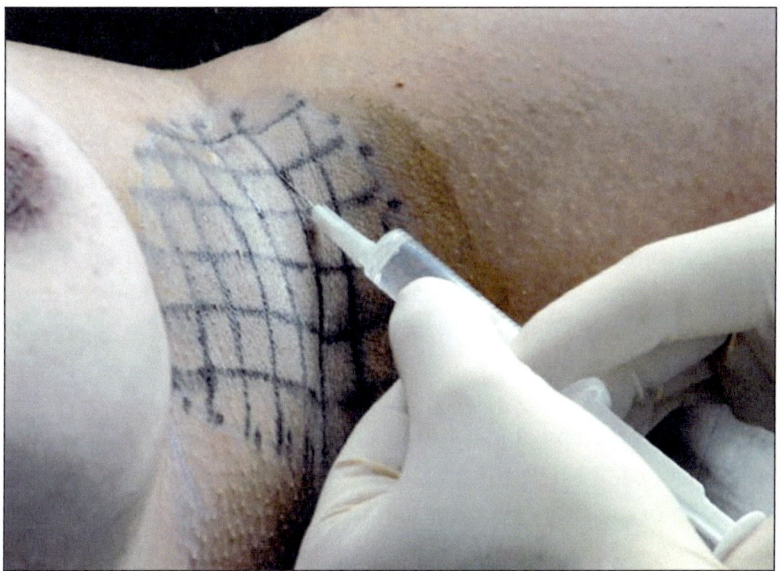

Fig. 9   Zonal division of the hyperhidrotic area with subsequent axillary Botox injection.

The side effects of Botox® application include the painful course of the therapy. In a few cases, hematomas may appear in the region of the injections. If the injection is administered carelessly, the toxin may also weaken the muscles. Botox® is contraindicated during pregnancy and breastfeeding. The safety and efficacy of Botox® for the treatment of primary axillary hyperhidrosis has not been studied in children and juveniles under 18 years of age.

Besides the treatment of local hyperhidroses, the injection therapy with Botox® represents a highly effective procedure for the treatment of the Frey syndrome. This specific form of gustatory perspiration in the cheek area has already been described in connection with the phenomenon of pathological sweating in the first part of this book.

All conventional therapeutic methods, such as surgery, physical therapy or even pharmacological approaches have been found to be ineffective or very high in side effects for the indication of Frey syndrome, so that their application is not in a reasonable proportion to the disturbing symptoms.

The treatment with botulinum toxin, however, has proven itself as a new and almost side-effect-free therapy, and has also been found to be a highly user friendly and minimally invasive anticholinergic strategy for blocking gustatory perspiration. The risk of a side effect exists only in the formation of neutralizing antibodies upon repeated injection therapy with higher doses in shorter intervals. The therapy may also be painful.

In a clinical therapy study, it was shown for the first time that with a dosage of $3 \, \text{MU/cm}^2$ of Botox®-A a complete and reliable blocking of gustatory perspiration for an effect duration of one year could be achieved, whereby said dosage is recommended.

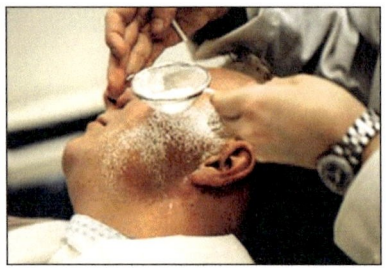 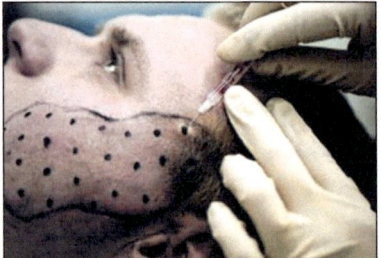

Fig. 10   Iodine-starch test in Frey-syndrome.

Fig. 11   Botox® injections in the hyperhidrotic half of the face.

As in the above-described Botox treatment for local hyperhidrosis, the perspiring skin part of the cheeks of the patient were first identified with the iodine-starch test after gustatory stimulation of sweat secretion by having the patient eat an apple. The stimulated sweating area was marked and cleaned. Then a punctiform marking with a spacing of 1 cm was made followed by the injections.

For this indication, a healing attempt was made, which is not yet listed in the service catalog of the health insurance due to the lack of controlled studies and for which therefore there is still no legal permission (Germany, status May 2005.)

7.2 Surgical removal of the sweat glands

Before patients and doctors consider a radical neurosurgical operation frequently accompanied by unforeseeable risks and side effects to relieve local hyperhidrosis, it should first be investigated whether milder surgical procedures may be indicated.

In this case, there is an alternative and less dangerous (in terms of possible adverse secondary symptoms) operation for the treatment of hyperhidrosis that is difficult to treat by conventional means, which is especially suitable if botulinum toxin is contraindicated.

In this surgical procedure, the sweat glands occurring in large numbers and high density in the armpit zone and responsible for the elevated secretion are removed.

This procedure is used in bromhidrosis, because the surgical removal of the apocrine sweat glands responsible for the odor in the armpit region promises a significant improvement (primarily used in Asia.)

Previously, the axillary skin regions were opened surgically and the glands then excised. This now obsolete procedure served for radical or partial excision of the sweat glands. Today, a glandular excision is still performed only in very persistent cases, and if at all, usually in combination with the newer procedures. The therapeutic effect of an excision is long lasting, although the patient must take considerable, above all, esthetic limitations in the bargain due to large area scarring and possible postoperative complications.

The older technique of patent removal of the glands has in the meanwhile been replaced by effective and continually optimized procedures such as subcutaneous sweat gland curettage or the increasingly more widely adopted sweat gland suction curettage or liposuction (more precisely: aspiration hidrectomy.) Liposuction, in particular, is an optimal surgical form of treatment in terms of the persistence of the therapeutic effect, the minor complications, side effects, and small scar size, as well as the possibility of repeating the operation, for normalization of local sweat secretion. In this combined procedure of curettage and liposuction, the glands and some of the fibers of the autonomic nervous system leading to them are removed. The more radical this removal is, the greater the therapeutic effect.

Liposuction, which will be discussed below, is a minimally invasive operation from the field of esthetic-cosmetic surgery that is indicated exclusively in the presence of a pronounced axillary hyperhidrosis or bromhidrosis. This procedure has recently attracted increased therapeutic interest because of its minimally invasive character.

It is also true of this procedure, which is now performed in many countries according to different standards, that it should be used only in specialized centers with a demonstrably large group of patients. The technical details of this operation vary and are of decisive importance for its success.

Aspiration hidrectomy

Medical-surgical representation of aspiration hidrectomy presented by Dr. Popp, Licca Clinic, Augsburg, Germany, October 2005.

Aspiration hidrectomy is recommended as an alternative to botulinum toxin therapy or surgical sympathicus blockade for armpit sweat. This actually involves fat extraction in the armpit. Whereas, in the case of adiposity of hips and thighs or abdominal fat, the fatty tissue is selectively removed and, by means of modern methods (tumescence anesthesia, special cannula) one attempts to cause as little secondary damage as possible, the process is utilized in the treatment of armpit perspiration in that older (aggressive) cannula models are supposed to remove as many sweat glands as possible with the same method.

In the older method of gland removal, the skin in the armpit was either completely removed while still under full anesthesia and the wound had to heal slowly, or a large flap of skin was folded over the wound and trimmed/dressed from below. Both procedures sometimes resulted in extensive and ugly scars, which frequently also caused mobility limitations after shrinking.

As a further development of the method, a local anesthesia is now applied in the armpit. In this case, tumescence local anesthesia is applied, in which a large quantity of local anesthetic is introduced into the armpit and the skin is thereby lifted off the underlying armpit tissue. Subsequently, after the anesthetic sets in, two small incisions (approximately 0.5–0.8 cm) are made above and below the armpit into which a quite aggressive cannula with the opening facing upwards is inserted and scrapes along under the skin. At this time minimal amounts of fat are obtained, but, above all, the sweat glands lying in the transition zone between the dermis and the subdermal fatty tissue are removed. So as to be sure, I myself then scrape again with another instrument and finally again suction out any remaining loose tissue fragments.

It is therefore the same as in liposuction, except that the target tissue is actually different. Instead of fat cells, the axillary sweat glands are suctioned out with a special cannula. They do not regenerate.

We call this procedure, incorrectly in the medical sense, liposuction – simply because laypersons can thus understand it – the average layman does not understand the term "aspiration hidrectomy."

If one takes one's time, the operation takes about two to three hours, whereby the operative sequence includes: arrival, changing clothes, iodine-starch test and marking of the OP field, disinfection, tumescence local anesthesia, numbing time, aspiration hidrectomy, bandaging the wound.

After the OP one should take it easy for the rest of the day and in no event drive a car. During the post-OP days there may still be a little pain in the armpit. Most patients do not perceive this as burdensome. It is important to bandage well, so that the skin in the armpits is pressed gently onto the underlying tissue. This will prevent the formation of a seroma (accumulation of tissue fluid) and the scarring will be better. Brownish spots rarely form in the OP region.

During the suction process, fine tunnels are created in the tissue, which contract during the healing phase, which would inhibit freedom of movement. It is therefore important to stretch the armpits several times daily, so that the skin does not stick together in an accordion fold. In this way, an unattractive armpit and a possible terminal limitation of movement are avoided.

To date I have encountered no serious problems with this OP. The patients tolerate the intervention and possible side effects well. It should be mentioned that the relapse rate is clearly higher than with the old method. However, in view of the advantages of suction, relapse should be accepted as part of the deal. If necessary, a follow-up operation is performed.

During the past 5 years I have not performed a single large-area excision of armpit sweat glands. Aspiration hidrectomy is certainly not my most frequently performed operation, but the tendency is clearly increasing; apparently the advantages are being communicated among patients and colleagues.

7.3 Sympathicolysis

Computed tomograph-(CT) controlled sympathicolysis is a relatively simple-to-perform therapy that may be considered after exhaustion of conservative measures for local hyperhidrosis cases (hands, feet, armpits, or for combined hyperhidrosis.)

In this outpatient procedure, with the aid of an imaging technique (CT), the sweat-controlling sympathic nerves are blocked by injection of a drug (sympathicolytic). The problem with this puncture operation, which has been characterized as minimally invasive, is the only temporary duration of the effect of the ganglion blockade, since regeneration of the blocked sympathic fibers is assumed. The therapeutic effect of reduced perspiration after sympathicolysis, depending on individual conditions, may range from only a few weeks up to several years. Because of this limitation, sympathicolysis is normally not included in the therapy plan for hyperhidrosis. In addition, the treatment of hyperhidrosis is not one of the primary indications for CT-supported sympathicolysis.

In the blockade procedure, the sympathic nerve blockade is performed in the region of the thoracic or lumbar vertebral column. Depending on the procedure, one speaks of thoracic or lumbar sympathicolysis. The thoracic procedure is chiefly considered for the treatment of local hyperhidrosis. In the case of hand and face sweating, the blockade of the T2 sympathic trunk is indicated, in the case of axillary hyperhidrosis, blockade of the T3 ganglion. A lumbar operation is performed if hyperhidrosis plantaris is present.

In clinical practice, with the patient in the abdominal position, after disinfection of the skin of the back in the region of the upper thoracic vertebrae under local anesthesia and CT monitoring, a fine puncture needle is inserted laterally next to the vertebral body. The cannula is then brought close to the sympathic ganglion under visual control in the CT device. There are several different techniques for the subsequent injection process. By successively injecting the sympathicolytic mixed with a contrast agent, the distribution of the drug mixture can be accurately monitored and corrected if necessary by repositioning the needle. Phenol is the preferred injection medium (a subject of controversy in the literature) since it causes fewer problems than an alcohol blockade (96% alcohol,) such as, e.g., nerve inflammations.

The syringe is then removed and a skin patch applied. The operation is performed ambulatorily, so that the patient can leave the clinic after a few hours of observation.

Depending on the region of the spinal column where the injection is performed, damage may occur to other structures during the operation. If the injection is through the thoracic space (in the case of hand sweating,) injuries to the pleura and lungs are possible. Harm to the kidneys or urinary tract by an operation in the lumbar vertebral region (in the case of plantar hyperhidrosis) is practically excluded, because the process is CT-supported. However, erectile and ejaculatory functional disorders may appear as a side effect. As with any other injection, side effects such as bleeding, infections, or nerve lesions may also occur in CT-controlled sympathicolysis. Also, a risk factor exists due to the radiation load related to the CT.

It has been described in the literature that the success rate of the endoscopic sympathicus blockade can be estimated on the basis of the sympathicolysis. Therefore, a sympathicolysis is frequently performed before this essentially irreversible operation, the latter being presented in detail in the following. However, the surgical nerve blockade is somewhat impeded by scar formation after a sympathicolysis, and therefore one should carefully consider which treatment appears indicated, in order to achieve an optimal therapeutic result.

7.4 Endoscopic sympathicus blockade

Probably the most radical solution for suppressing excessive perspiration is a surgical operation on the nerve ganglia of the autonomic nervous system that are responsible for controlling the sweat glands. By such an operation the predominantly sympathically controlled neuronal connections with the sweat glands are electrically blocked by transection, partial removal or compression, so that the sweat gland activity is reduced in the skin areas affected by the excessive perspiration. The surgical procedure of nerve transection is called a sympathicotomy, that of partial removal a sympathectomy. The minimally invasive keyhole technique commonly used today has changed the name of the process to "endoscopic transthoracic sympathectomy" (ETS). The compression blockade of the nerve structures, usually by applying metal clips, expanded the abbreviation to ETSC (C for clipping.) Generally, in the event of a blockade of nerve impulses of the sympathic nervous system, one can also speak of an "endoscopic sympathicus blockade" (abbreviation: ESB.) These designations and abbreviations are unfortunately not uniformly applied and sometimes supplemented by imaginative abbreviations.

The indication for an ETS(C)/ESB has long been confined to regional hyperhidroses on hands (hyperhidrosis manuum,) on the face (hyperhidrosis facialis,) and, in combination with the hands, in the armpits (hyperhidrosis axillaris.) Since the sympathic nervous system also includes the fibers of vascular control, the reddening of the facial skin also constitutes an indication for ETS(C)/ESB. Although this process, especially in cases of hyperhidrosis of the hands, due to the certainty of enduring, success, has been found to be superior to all other procedures of hyperhidrosis therapy, it is nevertheless linked to risks and side effects.

Such an operation should be applied only if extreme states of sweating are present which are experienced by the subject as burdensome for the health and limit the quality of life. If the indication is incorrect, the treated person may suffer seriously harmful and irreversible effects. Before hyperhidrotics subject themselves to such a therapeutic operation, they should consider meticulously, against the background of the potential risks, whether such a procedure is adequately proportional to their situation of suffering. The surgeon performing the treatment should also clearly inform the patients of the existing risks and possible consequences, despite the success rates that have demonstrably been achieved by sympathicus blockade.

The surgical procedure is not harmless and should therefore only be included as a last resort in the possible treatments for hyperhidrosis. Only when a hyperhidrotic has already completely exhausted nonsurgical therapeutic possibilities, such as externa (externally applied agents,) current treatment (iontophoresis,) and possible drug therapies without recognizable results, and intensive pressure of suffering persists, can the possibility of such an operation be taken into consideration. Complementary psychotherapeutic treatment should also be considered.

The technique of sympathicus blockade has been steadily improved, revised, and made more patient tolerable by the revolutionary results of endoscopic medicine. Thus, the traditional procedure of sympathectomy, in which the concealed nerve ganglia had to be exposed by painstaking surgical incisions (thoracotomy) is now considered obsolete and unreasonably burdensome for the patients. Currently, patients can be provided with a fundamentally modernized form of this technique whose practical application will be illustrated in the following within the scope of an experience report.

Due to the modern technique of endoscopy, we can reach the nerve ganglia in the thorax without complicated incisions and the inherent high risks for the patient. This modification of the sympathicus blockade is characterized medically as a minimally invasive operation that can be performed easily due to microendoscopy and which promises a high rate of success.

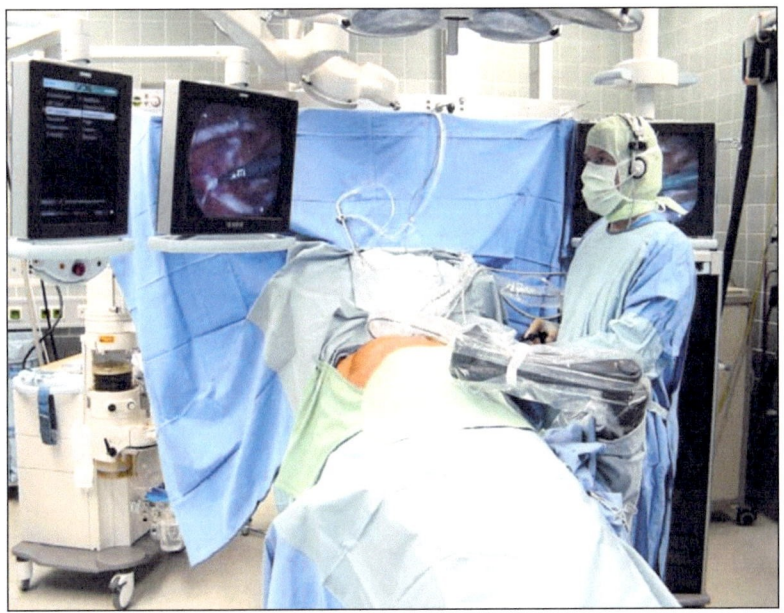

Fig. 12 Surgery situation of ETS.

The process is preferably used to relieve heavy sweating of the hands, armpits, and face. With the patient under general anesthesia, the surgeon, by means of small incisions in the chest wall and axillary cavity, creates an endoscopic access to the interior of the body. A special surgical endoscope is inserted into the body and permits the user to locate the ganglia responsible for the hyperperspiration in question.

These nerve structures are then blocked by the above-mentioned procedure. The operation is performed on each side for a symmetrical result. Only small, less than 1-cm-long, visible surgical scars remain. The patients can usually be discharged shortly after the operation.

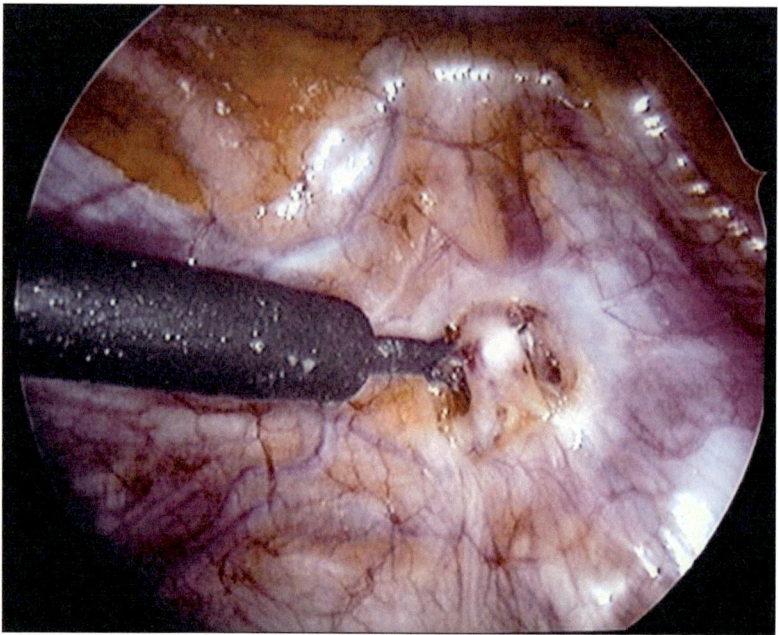

Fig. 13 Endoscopic photograph of the exposed ganglion.

Since every surgical operation involves risks and since changes result from any operation, the possible risks and side effects of this operation will be discussed here. Among the genuine risks of the sympathicus operation intercostal neuralgias, pain sensations in the thorax and shoulders, which arise due to the pressure of the instruments that are inserted between the ribs, must be mentioned. The miniaturization of surgical tools, however, has minimized these risks almost to zero. Persisting sensory disturbances or even symptoms of paralysis can hardly occur if the surgical technique is correct and should rather be regarded as therapeutic errors.

The so-called Horner syndrome and pneumothorax are among the dreaded complications of the thoracic sympathicus blockade, but they rarely occur when the patients are in the hands of experienced surgeons. The Horner syndrome occurs after injury of the uppermost thoracic ganglion and leads to a drooping eyelid and a constricted pupil. Although keenness of vision is not affected, a Horner syndrome signifies a relevant cosmetic change that can only be partially corrected. An injury to the pleural membrane covering the lungs causes air to escape from the lungs into the chest cavity (pneumothorax) and must be treated by thoracic drainage, a drain tube with suction fitting, for several days.

However, serious side effects are rarely observed. After the operation a reflexive increase in sweating occurs in the untreated areas of the body, which is called "compensatory sweating." This term is misleading since it promotes the belief that the quantity previously perspired on the hands, for example, has now been forced to be sweated out, for example, on the back. This sounds plausible, but, in fact, it is traceable to the blocking of the control system as a result of the operation. This effect occurs in all patients after the operation and must be discussed in detail beforehand. This phenomenon is usually described as tolerable in view of the later relief from sweating, but it can be very disturbing. The sweat pattern existing before the operation is of decisive importance. Patients with a not only regional but also whole-body "generalized" hyperhidrosis should not undergo a sympathicus blockade.

Depending on what technique is used for what indication, the operation may be accompanied by other adverse side effects. For example, because of the neuronal rearrangement, a postoperative reaction may be manifested in the form of gustatory sweating, which may be a new counterproductive burden for the patient, because the avoidance of sweating was the goal of the therapy. This gustatory perspiration or taste sweating is triggered via the sympathicus antagonist, the parasympathicus, and occurs primarily in the head-throat-neck region upon consumption of spicy or sour foods and beverages. Since the corresponding nerve structures cannot be blocked, the possibilities of treatment for this effect are limited.

The fibers leading toward the heart, which have a stimulating effect on the heart, are also blocked by the sympathicus blockade, so that the pulse and blood pressure are usually lower after the operation. This is often perceived as a pleasant side effect.

The different procedures used for ETS(C)/ESB are the subject of controversy in this context. Thus, against the background of the obligate compensatory sweating, the question arises of which nerve structures and segments should be blocked and which methods yield the best results. With regard to the most modern form of blockade, the nerve compression by metal clips, the question as to what extent the nerves recover after removal of the clips has also not yet been adequately researched.

The association of the *International Society for Sympathetic Surgery* to which ETS surgeon, private lecturer Dr. Christoph Schick, director of the German Hyperhidrosis Center DHHZ in Munich belongs as chairman, is concerned with the scientific development of ETS(C)/ESB. According to Dr. Schick, there is currently no final classification or treatment plan with respect to surgical sympathicus blockade. Nevertheless, there are some clear therapy techniques that have found widespread application. Thus, one should basically proceed as minimalistically as possible, i.e., the extent of the blockade should be confined to the region of heaviest perspiration and avoid extensive destruction and partial removal of the nerves. The sympathic ganglion is not a simple point-to-point connection but rather to be understood as the "backbone" of a network into which the impulses of several vertebral levels enter and exit again by different routes. For all areas of the body, however, there are "conduction levels" by which most of the nerve impulses flow into the system. For the head, this is the T2 level, for the hands T3, and for the armpits T4.

According to Dr. Schick, more recent results indicate that a blockade of the nerve branches is just as effective as the switching off of the ganglia (nerve nodes) themselves, that the use of compression clips (titanium clips) yields results as good as transection, and that deeper nerve blockades tend to cause less pronounced side effects than higher ones. Therefore, he recommends a blockade of the corresponding conduction levels by using clips without impairing the ganglia. In his view, the correct indication is also of decisive importance. His many years of research have shown, for example, that excessive sweating on the trunk existing before and as the main reason for the operation (generalized hyperhidrosis) results in a considerably stronger "compensatory" sweating with clearly reduced patient satisfaction. In his opinion, as there is no benefit, these patients should not be subjected to the operation, he has therefore developed an elaborate method for quantifying the sweating on the different parts of the body and for setting up an individual sweat pattern profile. According to Dr. Schick, this measurement is indispensable before an operation, because many patients do not subjectively perceive their dynamic sweating pattern.

Unfortunately, in the field of ETS(C)/ESB, progress is slow, bearing in mind that new evidence can only be acquired by very costly studies following scientific principles. Moreover, the patients are widely geographically scattered, so that a consistent scientific follow-up scarcely seems possible.

The well-known ETS surgeon Dr. Ivo Tarfusser of Italy, who has performed the treatment since the end of the 1980s and has a population with more than 1800 interventions, asserts that patients from a large number of countries (including Australia, New Zealand, Canada, USA, Viet Nam, and China) have undergone a surgical sympathicus blockade. Professional ETS(C)/ESB surgery is now also available in these countries.

Sympathicus surgery

Trends in sympathicus surgery presented by Dr. Tarfusser, Meran, Italy, November, 2005.

A high-[level] interruption (between Th1 and Th2 or an exclusion of the Th2 ganglion) tends towards a less favorable side effect spectrum than a lower interruption (below the Th2 ganglion.)

The consequences may be stronger compensatory sweating to the point of compensatory hyperhidrosis, a stronger damping of the circulation to the point of lower blood pressure (in individual cases,) bradycardia or fatigue.

Such a high interruption is therefore no longer performed by some surgeons (myself included) for hand sweating. In the case of head sweating or erythema, however, one usually has no alternative, and the ganglion must be interrupted above Th2.

Of all states in which a surgical sympathicus blockade is applied, craniofacial hyperhidrosis (sweating on the face) entails the greatest risk of development of compensatory hyperhidrosis. In my statistics, 12% of the patients operated on who had facial sweating wished they could reverse the operation (removal of the clips.)

For comparison, in patients with erythrophobia (fear of blushing,) the clips were removed in 6.5% of the cases, while for hand sweating, only in exceptionally rare cases (<1%.)

A point of debate that is still not officially clarified is whether the use of the clamping method (neurocompression, clipping) with titanium clips is really reversible. Admittedly, a corresponding study can only be performed with extreme difficulty and thus every surgeon pursues his/her own path.

I am personally convinced that the nerve can recover upon removal of the clip under favorable conditions, whereby many details are of importance, such as the pressure exerted on the nerve (avoiding pinching,) the diameter of the nerve, pre-existing anatomic conditions, clip material, duration of compression, etc.

In my experience, more than two thirds of the patients in whom clips were removed report a distinct improvement of the compensatory sweating after 6–12 months.

Unfortunately, there is no control group for an objective evaluation and no objective methods of measurement, for which reason the results must be considered with the necessary restraint from a strictly scientific standpoint.

Personally, I still prefer the clamp method and perform a complete separation only in case of recurrence and upon urgent request on the part of the patient.

For cases of hand sweating, I prefer isolation (clamping above and below, or the ramus communicans) of the Th3 ganglion, with the result of less compensatory sweating and other side effects than in the case of Th2 (with at least an equally good result and better results than with the Th4 method.)

The method is slowly gaining more and more followers. As a variant, the simple interruption between Th2 and Th3 is often performed; the future will show whether or the relapse rate also increases as a result.

It is still important to have a correct and restrictive indication (strong impairment due to hyperhidrosis and failure of conservative methode,) which in some cases was perhaps not taken into account and provided the media with negative headlines.

A patient's experience

Whoever suffers from hyperhidrosis – whatever the form – knows how great the emotional burden is that a patient must bear. I myself suffered from hyperhidrosis facialis (facial sweating.) Toward the end, only the smallest trigger was necessary. A discussion with a salesperson in a department store or supermarket became torture, the change from cold weather outside to a warm room, birthday parties, simple visits to bars, and even going to the movies were almost impossible. Every time I started dripping from the face.

After 6 years of suffering I decided for the first time to look for information about the sweat problem on the Internet. At this point, I still didn't know that I was actually sick, but had nearly always disregarded the causes of the sweating and morbidly focused on the night sweating. However, the more I tried not to sweat, the more sweat flowed – which is not news to anyone.

It was just one big vicious circle. In my hyperhidrosis, about 70% of the cause was emotional. In the Internet, I somehow found a site on hyperhidrosis. This was my salvation, as I now know.

In a discussion forum, I made my first call in the hope that someone could explain to me what kind of a disease I actually have. Even today I am impressed by how many responses I received, how kindly my questions were answered and how much detailed advice was given. From then on I knew: You are not alone! I was just glad that I could exchange information with others.

I was finally informed of an operation, the ETS. I gathered information and constantly encountered the name of Dr. Tarfusser as a respected surgeon specializing in this field. I got addresses, telephone numbers and a lot of info, until I decided one day to simply call Dr. Tarfusser.

I also immediately set a date for this ETS, being very well aware that this is the last step to be taken. However, the pressure of my suffering was so great that I saw no other options. The date of surgery was soon agreed, within some 3 weeks my operation would take place in Meran, Italy. I had my family doctor send the EKG requested by Dr. Tarfusser and had my blood count determined. To be on the safe side, I also had an examination for a malfunction of the thyroid gland. Thus far the short version of my pre-OP case history.

Meran, Italy, May 23, 2001 at Dr. Ivo Tarfusser's

The ETS deadline on May23, 2001 grew closer and closer... Then I found myself at 9 a.m. on the morning of the date of the operation fasting in the St. Anna Clinic in Meran. As before every operation, after midnight no food or drinks could be taken. Dr. Tarfusser discussed my previous diseases with me. He questioned me once more in great detail about the form and intensity of my hyperhidrosis.

Then he explained to me in detail the various surgical methods (cut and clamping) and informed me of the possible risks of the operation (above all, the compensatory sweating, the so-called Horner syndrome was said to be almost excluded nowadays.) During this discussion I also became acquainted with the anesthesiologist, Dr. Friedrich, and together we filled out a questionnaire on anesthesia. Both Dr. Tarfusser and Dr. Friedrich made a calming, friendly and very competent impression on me. This relieved a great part of my concerns.

A few minutes later I was given the OP gown and the thrombosis stockings. I had to undress completely and put them both on. Then I was taken in my bed one floor lower to the operating room antechamber. There, I got up and was escorted into the operating room itself by Dr. Friedrich. I lay down on the operating table, had a pair of electrodes connected to my back, and then my arms were fastened away from my body by special holders. The armpits were supposed to be shaved in advance, but, in my case, this was no longer necessary. Dr. Friedrich then inserted the infusion needle on the back of my right hand, administered at first two small infusions, and then the anesthetic. He had scarcely told me that I would fall asleep any minute now when I already entered dreamland.

Operation report

Operation: Endoscopic transthoracic interganglionic sympath-ecotomy Th1-2 bilaterally, May 23, 2001.
Surgeon: Dr. Ivo Tarfusser, Anesthesiologist: Dr. Friedrich

Intubation anesthesia Centimeter-long incision in the left armpit and blunt preparing of the subcutaneous channel up to the 3rd rib in the anterior axillary line. The Verres needle is inserted at the upper edge of the 3rd rib into the pleural cavity. After insufflation of 2 liters of CO2, the resectoscope is inserted into the thoracic cavity, lesions on the lung surface excluded, and the sympathic ganglion identified. Fenestration of the pleura and severance of the ganglion well below the ganglion stellatum at the upper limit of the 2nd rib with clean cutting current of low intensity. The Kuntze collateral nerve is thereby spared, in order to permit medium-term sympathic reinnervation of the palms if necessary. Removal of the endoscope after aspiration of the CO_2 and closure of the incision with intracutaneous Vicryl rapid. Following this, an identical procedure is performed on the right half of the thorax. Operation completely free of complications.

A few minutes after the complication-free operation that lasted 50 minutes I woke up in the recovery room. To my surprise, I did not have these pains on my sternum many others have reported. Even the surgical wounds did not hurt. They were covered with a water-impermeable transparent special bandage.

At around 6:30 a.m. the next morning, my blood pressure and temperature were measured again. In the meanwhile I felt quite well, even the mild breathing problems occurring throughout the night were tolerable. Around 8 o'clock Dr. Tarfusser visited me again. We spoke for the last time about the operation, and before my release he reminded me to phone him in a few weeks.

Postoperative experience

06/11/2001

Some 3 weeks after my operation I have to say that in the meantime things have gone very well. I haven't sweated on my head once in situations unpleasant for me. My forehead was always absolutely dry! Restaurant visits and birthdays were real relief! As before, I may still sweat on my head during sports! Not especially a lot, but my forehead does become slightly moist to wet. That is very good and important! My resting pulse is a little slower. I no longer have any pain. The surgery wounds have healed nicely on both sides and are scarcely visible.

The compensatory sweating has stabilized somewhat, although it is still different from day to day. Above all, I now sweat more on the legs (mostly on my shins.) Also a bit on the back and stomach, but it doesn't worry me.

11/01/2005

After the operation more than 4 years ago, I have noticed the following changes in health. The head sweating has been eliminated by about 95%, the other pathological sweating symptoms I had, too. I still sweat on the forehead when engaging in sports. Dripping wet only in summer (but never more than others, rather less,) but this stops very quickly as soon as I take a break. Therefore, everything in the green! When the thermometer in summer reads 35°C, then I sweat lightly on the forehead, just like other people!

The compensatory sweating (CS) has improved since my ETS. It is still present, but the condition has become tolerable. If before I sweated very heavily for even the slightest reason, then this is now only the case in highly emotional situations, in which I used to turn beet red and sweated extremely on the face. At such moments my back and stomach become a little damp. In very warm rooms it still happens that I get wet in these regions, but this is scarcely noticed by others. Even these situations in which I get CS have become fewer because I am generally more at ease. Sultry weather (~30°C in the summer and high humidity) is a horror for every ETS-person, and the CS is also annoying then (back and abdomen may but do not always have to get wet, sometimes also the shins.) Nevertheless, I manage quite well and it doesn't represents a major problem.

My terrible blushing (which I always had before the operation) has almost entirely disappeared! Once in a blue moon I may feel my cheeks turn red in unpleasant situations, but no one notices, and perhaps I am only imagining it. I also don't think about it any more. The reddening in the case of prolonged stays in warm rooms occurs now and then. Before or after drinking alcohol I get bright red and hot cheeks, but it actually doesn't bother me much.

Overall balance

Positive aspects:

- 95% elimination of facial sweating
- 90% elimination of blushing
- Resting pulse, once 75 bpm lowered to approx. 60 bpm, so that during athletics there is usually an exercise pulse of only 150, no more, which is not at all bad
- physical performance capacity absolutely positive, no changes compared to before the ETS
- generally more "inner peace" in all everyday situations
- enormously strengthened self-esteem
- no observable "sexual disfunctions" that are often discussed as side effects in many Internet forums

Negative aspects

- the compensatory sweating, although this improved with time. At first it was hard to tolerate, but now it is within absolutely tolerable limits

- rarely dry eyes, but I am not sure whether this is really related to the ETS

- mild-to-medium gustatory sweating (on the forehead) and slight blushing (cheeks become slightly red) when eating spicey dishes (with a lot of curry, pepper, chili, pepperoni) and some fruits (plums,) and within limits when eating "nutella" and similar chocolate crèmes – also a type of "goose bumps" when eating these dishes

Personal conclusion:

I am immensely content since my ETS more than 4 years ago. The more than 6000 DM ($ 3500) I paid at that time were well invested; I have never regretted it. If such an operation were necessary again, I would have it done again.

Against the background of expanded therapy options for the indication of hyperhidrosis inspires hope for the future. Possibly, neurotoxins with longer-lasting effect and alternative remedies will soon be in use, in order to treat hyperhidrosis even more effectively. New findings in the not yet fully researched chemical transport mechanisms in the epidermis that are essentially responsible for the sweat gland activation process may disclose additional and alternative therapeutic possibilities, which may perhaps soon permit surgery to be avoided.

Finally, it should be stressed once more that therapy for hyperhidrosis belongs exclusively in professional hands and must be administered in cooperation with a medical specialist. Medically objectionable self-medication, especially with drugs from the group of anticholinergics or psychopharmaceuticals, is strictly inadvisable.

8. Cost coverage by health insurance

A topic frequently discussed by patients is the question of whether the cost of operations will be covered and the medications prescribed for treatment of hyperhidrosis will be paid for. Binding statements on this subject are possible only conditionally, especially since the question of cost coverage comes under the state-specific regulations and depends on the public health laws, the national coverage system in question, and, ultimately, the insurance status of the individual. While many medications and drugs can generally be prescribed depending on their legal status, in the case of the surgical measures under consideration here, problems often arise for patients as well as therapists, since coverage is a decision made by the insurer.

After the diagnosis of hyperhidrosis is made and the symptoms described, as a rule, the classic stepwise therapy is instituted. An absolute prerequisite here is the exhaustion of conventional therapeutic options. If they all remain without effect, then it is necessary to document medically the therapeutic necessity of the next treatment within the framework of the stepwise plan.

Patients should follow this approach in the event of problems with insurance, always in consultation with their therapist. The latter has the necessary competence and will prepare the required reports on the previous therapeutic course and the prospects of success of the desired/requested therapy, as well as correspond with the insurance carrier. He can also refer to the serious mental consequences of hyperhidrosis, the impairment of the quality of life in the workplace and in social life that would certainly result in additional and higher costs in the event of refusal. That the insurer pay the costs is better achieved in this way, rather than by the patient's attempting it alone. Moreover, the therapists in most cases already have ready-to-use forms and petitions for cost coverage, especially concerning many of the scientifically recognized therapies, such as iontophoresis or Botox injection. Especially in the case of the classic therapy of iontophoresis, experience shows that, when the therapeutic instructions are followed, there are fewer problems in financing the therapy than in the case of surgery.

Some applications have no legally licensed indication for therapy of hyperhidrosis, although their effectiveness has long been proven in extensive research. Most insurers, taking into consideration the cost explosion in the public health system, will first attempt to deny coverage in such cases.

The use of drugs and applications is limited to certain fields of application. In the case of application outside of the license, one speaks of "off-label use." Off-label use is the use of licensed treatment methods or drugs for another purpose than described in the user information (package insert) or technical information for the remedy or of unlicensed drugs.

Basically, the performance obligation of the insurers is limited to the fields of application named in the drug license.

The prescription of a drug in an unlicensed field of application is permissible when the treatment of a serious disease is involved, no other therapy is available, and when, based on the available data, the prospect exists that therapeutic success can be achieved with the preparation. In order for the insurer to be obliged to perform, all three conditions must be satisfied.

The patient is advised to document in detail all previously attempted approaches, drugs prescribed, doctor and clinic visits, and unsuccessfully applied therapies, in order to have them available in the case of subsequent treatments and to have them available at any time for forthcoming process decisions. Depending on insurance status, it should also be clarified whether besides or instead of legal health insurance, private or additional insurance would cover the costs of the treatment.

In the introduction to this book, the development of the Internet was described as a revolutionary advance for the diagnosis and therapy of hyperhidrosis. However, the Internet and its free accessibility also represent a not to be underestimated risk for the patient. The free availability and unlimited access, especially to prescription-requiring drugs conceals great dangers, and many patients who out of shame do not wish to discuss their problem with a therapist are tempted to try self-medication. In most cases, no one assumes responsibility for the correctness of the information on the Internet. Manufacturer and seller often even remain unacknowledged and act purely for profit reasons. Even drugs with a high addiction potential can be delivered to your home without problems.

Therefore, this method must be strictly advised against, because it lacks the necessary preliminary extensive examination, diagnosis, and qualified counseling by a doctor. Unprofessional self-medication without accurate knowledge of the drug may have incalculable consequences for the health and safety standards corresponding to the drug laws of the states cannot be guaranteed.

The wrongful taking of drugs and spoiled, adulterated, overdosed or underdosed medications may lead to serious impairment of health. The important patient information pamphlets are often difficult to understand, written in a foreign language, or totally missing. Possible side effects are not always reported and warnings, e.g., of the risk of drug dependence, are frequently lacking.

9.   Concluding remarks and references

Now that you, dear reader, have almost reached the end of this adviser, you will have gained insight into the complexity of causes, symptoms, and therapy forms of the disease called hyperhidrosis.

In the first part of the book, your attention was directed to the multiple causes found both in the physical and also in the psychological realm.

Inasmuch as you yourself are afflicted by excessive perspiration, you will have acquired the knowledge that this set of symptoms can be effectively treated and that its sufferers need no longer be victims of this pathological state. As was shown in the second part of the book, numerous therapeutic approaches now exist for effectively countering an nonphysiologically caused sweat secretion.

In the first edition of this book, the lack of information sources concerning this topic was lamented. Today, a good 5 years after the first edition, the information situation on the subject of hyperhidrosis has been fundamentally changed.

International self-help groups, discussion forums, and special-interest groups have been established on the Internet. For many of the afflicted, it is a relief to know that there are other people with the same health problems. Via the Internet, the person seeking advice is able benefit from the countless reports and recommendations of those afflicted with this condition.

This world-spanning medium, however, also contains considerable dangers. Since the Internet is not subject to a controlling authority, serious and technically competent material may stand totally free of judgment beside subjective experience reports and even dangerous suggestions or totally false advice. One needs to be very watchful and filter out the correct information.

It is precisely the commercial aspects which lead many dealers to make a "quick buck" from the misfortune of the afflicted. For this reason, we must especially warn against costly surgical procedures not covered by insurance for relieving pathological sweating. Such operations are often claimed to be the only therapeutic possibility. The experiences of many former sufferers show that this is not so.

The well-informed patient should apply longsightedness here and first subject his (co)decision as to what therapeutic route to follow to a thorough study of the variety of help offered.

In the following, data from the literature and contact addresses are listed. In addition, some websites are listed which are concerned with the topic of pathological perspiration in a special way and, in the view of the author and many patients, merit the term "helpful." This book is also accompanied by an Internet project. At the website **www.transpiration.de** supplements to the subjects discussed here and further services concerning this topic are presented.

References

Literature and reference works incorporated in this book were obtained for the most part from the following publications. They may serve the interested reader as reference works.

Achten, B., Ratgeber Starkes Schwitzen – was tun? Nordmark Arznei-mittel GmbH 1994

Achenbach, R. K., Schwitzen. Ein Ratgeber für Gesunde und Betroffene, Kybermed GmbH & Co, 2000

Achenbach, R. K., Hyperhidrosis. Physiologisches und krankhaftes Schwitzen in Diagnose und Therapie, Steinkopf 2004

Achenbach, R. K., Der Haut-Ratgeber, TRIAS '97

Drobik, **Laskawi**, **Schwab** (1995), Therapie des Frey-Syndroms mit Botulinum-Toxin. Erfahrungen mit einer neuen Behandlungsmethode. HNO 43: 644-648

Fidler, H. P., Der Schweiß, Entstehung, Zusammensetzung und Bekämp-fung, Aulendorf, Cantor, 1968

Heckmann, M., **Rzany**, B., Behandlung der fokalen Hyperhidrose. Botu-linumtoxin in der Dermatologie. Medizin und Wissen, München 2002, S. 53-75

Heckmann, M., **Breit**, S., **Ceballos-Baumann**, A., **Schaller**, M., **Ple-wig**, G., Axilläre Hyperhidrose: Erfolgreiche Behandlung mit Botu-linumtoxin-A, Hautarzt 1998; 49: 101-103

Heckmann, M., **Plewig**, G., Behandlung der Hyperhidrose mit Botulinum-toxin-A, Editorial auf Einladung der Redaktion des Deutschen Ärzte-blattes, gekürzte und revidierte Fassung M. Heckmann

Hilbrans, J., Die therapeutische Anwendung von Aluminiumchlorid-lösungen zur Behandlung der Hyperhidrosis axillaris, Univ. Düssel-dorf, Diss. 1990

Hilbrans, J., **Hölzle**, E., Die Behandlung der Hyperhidrosis axillaris mit Aluminiumchloridlösungen, Aktuelle Dermatologie, 20. Jg., 1994, S. 303-308

Hölzle, E., Antiperspiranzien – Wirkungsweise, Wirkungsprüfung und praktische Anwendung, Zeitschrift für die Körperpflegemittel-, Par-fümerie-, Riechstoff- und Aerosol-Industrie, 114. Jg., Nr. 7/88, S. 249-253

Hölzle, E. u. a., Die gepulste Gleichstrom-Iontophorese als neue Behand-lungsmöglichkeit der Hyperhidrosis, Hautarzt (1995) 46, S. 543-547, Springer Verlag

Hölzle, E., Axilläre und palmoplantare Hyperhidrosis, Dt. Ärzteblatt 85. Jg., Heft 44, S. 3055-3063, 1988

Hölzle, E., **Alberti**, N. (1987), Long-term efficacy and side effects of tap water iontophoresis of palmar hyperhidrosis – the usefulness of home therapy. Dermatologica 175: 126-1355

Kluth, S. M., Über die systemische Therapie der idiopathischen Hyperhidrosis generalisata, Univ. Düsseldorf, Diss. 1997

Kreyden, O. P., **Burg**, G., Hyperhidrosis and Botulinumtoxin in Dermatology (USA), S. Karger Publishers, 2002

Neues Rezept Formularium (NRF), Loseblattsammlung, Govi-Verlag

Nickel, J., **Jahnel**, A., **Andresen**, R., CT-gestützte lumbale Sympathikolyse bei Hyperhidrosis plantaris, RöFo 2004; 176: 1

Nolte, D., **Gollmitzer**, I., **Loeffelbein**, D. J., **Hölzle**, F., **Wolff**, K.-D., Botulinumtoxin zur Behandlung des gustatorischen Schwitzens. Eine prospektive randomisierte Therapiestudie, Mund Kiefer GesichtsChir 2004; 8: 369–375

Peros, I., Langzeitergebnisse nach subkutaner Schweißdrüsenkürettage bei Hyperhidrosis axillaris, Univ. Marburg, Diss. 1999

Plewig, G., **Nachbar**, F., **Blecher**, P., **Hüttenrauch**, C., Hyperhidrosis und Iontophorese. Nicht jedes Gerät wirkt gleich, Zt. für Dermatologie 181 (1995) Nr.1: 43-44

Plewig, G., **Jansen**, Th., Hyperhidrosis (Folge 2): Idiopathische Hyperhidrosis, Therapie, MMW-Fortschr.Med. 141 (1999): 498-499

Reinauer, S., **Schauf**, F., **Hubert**, M., **Hölzle**, E. (1992), Wirkungsmechanismus der Leitungswasser-Iontophorese: Funktionelle Störung des sekretorischen Epithels. Z Hautkr 67: 622-626

Reinauer, S., **Neußer**, A., **Schauf**, G., **Hölzle**, E. (1995), Die gepulste Gleichstrom-Iontophorese als neue Behandlungsmöglichkeit der Hyperhidrosis. Hautarzt 46: 543-547

Ruzicka, T., **Kohls-Zinnhobler**, I., Die Iontophoresebehandlung der Hyperhidrosis palmoplantaris, MMV 1990

Rzany, B., **Hund**, M. (2003), Fokale Hyperhidrosis. Hautarzt 54: 767-780

Schara, R., Die Therapie einer Hyperhidrosis mit einem Parkinsonmedikament, Therapiewoche 43, 23 (1993): 1374-1375

Sonntag, M., **Ruzicka**, T. (2005), Hyperhidrose – Ursachen und aktuelle Behandlungsmöglichkeiten, psychoneuro 2005; 31 (6): 315–320

Fuchslocher, M., **Rzany**, B., Orale anticholinerge Therapie der fokalen Hyperhidrose mit Methantheliniumbromid (Vagantin®.) Hautarzt 2002; 2: 151-152

Zittlau, J., Natürlich heilen mit Salbei, Ludwig, München 2000

Survey of medications

Listed below are the drugs for treatment of pathological perspiration. This survey was prepared with the aid of the most commonly consulted pharmaceutical indices (*Red and yellow drug list, Germany,*) based on experience reports of patients, and after consulting other specialty medical sources. They are intended to serve patients as an aid in orientation. This list is not to be considered exhaustive. Certain active principles are a component of a great variety of pharmaceutical preparations available on the market, all of which cannot be listed here. This survey does not replace an examination or diagnosis by a certified physician. Therefore any liability for the correctness and completeness of the information listed below is waived.

Therapeutic agents for treatment of hyperhidrosis belong to the indication group of dermatics from the pharmacological standpoint. However, in the treatment of hyperhidrosis, it is found that preparations with other indications, e.g., spasmolytics, antiseptics, gastro-intestinal remedies, sedatives, or hypnotics may lead to good therapeutic results. They are frequently prescribed for off-label use.

The following listing of drugs is according to trade name, form of administration, and active principle. It includes the drugs commonly mentioned in the literature in connection with hyperhidrosis. Various preparations are not licensed in some states or under other trade names or as generics, respectively. By stating the active principle, the possibility exists of searching for a pharmaceutical license for certain drugs also in other states.

Herbal antihidrotics[1]

Salbei Curarina®, drops, active ingredient: sage

Salbei Tropfen®, active ingredient: sage

Salus®, drops, active ingredient: sage

Sweatosan® N, pills, active ingredient: sage

Nosweat® N, capsules, active ingredient: sage leaf extract

Salvysat® Bürger, pills or solution, active ingredient: sage

Jaborandi Pentarkan® S, drops, homeopathic combination preparation

Pflügerplex® **Sambucus** 122, solution, homeopathic combination preparation

Salvia® **Oligoplex**, drops, homeopathic combination preparation

Anticholinergics -- Antihypertensives

Anticholinergics

Sormodren®, tablets, active ingredient: bornaprine

Vagantin®, pills, active ingredient: methanthelinum bromide

Atropinum® sulfuricum, tablets, active ingredient: atropine

Ditropan XL®, tablets, active ingredient: oxybutynin chloride

Pro-Banthine®, tablets, active ingredient: propantheline bromide

Belladonnysat® Bürger, juice or solution, active ingredient: belladonna alkaloids (see also hyoscyamine)

Robinul® **(Forte),** tablets, active ingredient: **g**lycopyrrolate

---

[1] Some of the drugs named contain alcohol. The homeopathic remedies listed have no unequivocal indication.

Receptor blockers

Inderal®, tablets, active ingredient: propranolol-HCl ß-receptor blocker

Propabloc®, tablets, active ingredient: propranolol-HCl ß-receptor blocker

Catapresan®, tablets, active ingredient: clonidine HCl (alpha-2-adrenoceptor agonist)

Clonidin-ratiopharm®, capsules, active ingredient: clonidine HCl (alpha-2-adrenoceptor agonist)

Clonistada®, tablets, active ingredient: clonidine HCl (alpha-2-adrenoceptor agonist)

Dermatics: Astringents – Antihidrotics

Alsol®, crème, active ingredient: aluminum acetate-tartrate

Essitol®, tablets, active ingredient: aluminum acetate-tartrate

Antihydral®, salve, active ingredient: methenamine

Tannolact®, crème, grease-crème, gel, lotion, powder, active ingredient: phenol-methanal-urea polycondensate, sulfonated

Ansudor® **(N)**, emulsion or powder, aluminum hydroxychloride, Triclocarban

Tannosynt®, crème, lotion, powder, active ingredient: phenol-methanal urea polycondensate, sulfonated, sodium salt (synthetic tannin)

Aluminum-chloride-based antiperspirants[2]

Indication Hyperhidrosis in part with antibacterial effect

Anhydrol Forte®, Driclor®, Certain Dri®, Odaban®, medisan+® Spray, Yerka® Deodorant Antiperspirant, Drysol®, Etiaxil®, Dehydral® Cream (Methenamine 8 %), Bionova®, 5-Day®, AHC®-Antiperspirant

Indication Bromhidrosis

Crystal Spray Body Deodorant™ (without aluminum chloride)
BromEx Foam® (on market after summer 2006, company JV Cosmetics)

Individual formulation of aluminum chloride solutions in alcohol or water:
– 15% variable (w/v) aluminum chloride hexahydrate ($AlCl_3$)
– 1% silicone oil
– ad 100 ml ethanol or aqua dest

Psychopharmaceuticals

Benzodiazepam

Valium®, tablets, active ingredient: diazepam

Antidepressives

Xanax®, tablets, active ingredient: alprazolam

Fluctin®, tablets, solution, capsules, active ingredient: fluoxetin

Herbal Psychopharmaceuticals

Baldrian-Dispert®, pills, active ingredient: Baldrian

Johanniskraut-ratiopharm®, capsules, drops, active ingredient: St. John's wort

---

[2] The therapeutic efficacy of the products named depends on the concentration of the active principle involved.

Botulinum toxin

Botox[®], injection, active ingredient Clostridium botulinum Toxin Type A 100 E, Pharm Allergan GmbH

Dysport[®], injection, active ingredient Clostridium botulinum Toxin Type A 500 U, Ipsen Pharma GmbH

More detailed information on the active principle botulinum toxin may be found on the website www.botulinumtoxin.de of the working group Botulinumtoxin of the German Society for Neurology.

Internet and contact addresses

Web pages are subject to constant changes. Therefore, it may occur that a domain or its contents are no longer current. At least in the pertinent forums on hyperhidrosis, however, one will always find information on the currently important developments and projects.

The contents of the Internet pages listed here are not my responsibility. I am only responsible for the contents of the home page accompanying this book www.transpiration.de.

Information pages in German

- **http://www.transpiration.de**
  Homepage of this book

- **http://www.hyperhidrosehilfe.de**
  The self help forum (+ shop) for people with sweating problems

- **http://www.psychic.de**
  Besides hyperhidrosis this deals with aspects of social phobia.

- **http:/www.schwitzfleck.at** (Austria)
  German-speaking hyperhidrosis community

International information pages

- **http://www.sweathelp.org** (USA, multilingual)
  The International Hyperhidrosis Society (IHHS) established in 2003 is a common interest organization for clarification and research on excessive sweating. Through its program the IHHS offers affected access to therapies and supports education and advanced training of physicians. The goal of the IHHS is the improvement of the life quality of those suffering hyperhidrosis.

- **http://www.parsec.it/summit/hyper1d.htm** (Italy)   Hyperhidrosis – excessive perspiration, Dr. Ivo Tarfusser

- **http://www.esfbchannel.com**
  Online community for patients

- **http://www.hyperhidrosisinfo.com**
  Page with extensive information

- **http://www.hyperhidrosiscenter.com**
  German Hyperhidrosis Center (DHHZ), Munich

Discussions forums

- **http://www.ctsnet.org** (USA)
  A lively international forum on hyperhidrosis, can be accessed via the home page – Click on Discussion

- **http://www.hh-forum.de** (Germany)
  German discussion forum Hyperhidrosis with chat

- **http://www.hyherhidrosehilfe.de** (Germany)
  Self-help forum (plus shop) for people with sweating problems

- **http://www.ets-talk.com** (USA)
  ETS And Reversals Discussion Forum. Discussions on endoscopic sympathectomy and its side effects

- **http://communities.msn.com/ExcessiveSweatHH/ bromboard.msn**
  Bromhidrosis Board, discussion forums on Hyperhidrosis and Bromhidrosis

International information sources and surgeons

- **http://www.suor.com.br** (Brazil)
  Dr. Peter Kux and Dr. João Bosco Vieira Duarte

- **http://www.parsec.it/summit/hyper1d.htm** (Italy) Dr. Ivo Tarfusser

- **http://www.hyperhidrosis.de** (Germany)
  Dr. Christoph Schick

- **http://www.privatix.fi** (Finland)
  Dr. Telaranta, Dr. Lin

- **http:/www.sweaty-palms.com** (USA)
  The Center for Hyperhidrosis – A cure for excessive sweating by Dr. Reisfeld

- **http://www.handsdry.com** (USA)
  The Hyperhidrosis Center by Dr. Jim Garza

- **http:/www.hyperhidrosis.com** (worldwide)
  Internationale Ärztevereinigung – Surgical Team

- **http://www.handsweat.com** (USA)
  American Institute for Hyperhidrosis by Dr. Kenneth Adam Lee, Dr. Leon Egozi

- **http://www.hyperhidrosisusa.com** (USA)
  Dr. David Nielson

Contact addresses

The following contact addresses are also listed on the homepage accompanying this book. The author is making every effort to keep it updated.

Iontophoresis therapy

Hidrex GmbH

Otto-Hahn-Str. 12, D-42579 Heiligenhaus
Tel.: +49 (0)2 056/256481, Fax: +49 (0)2 056/257743
Service Hotline: +49 (0)1805/981100
http://www.hidrex.de, E-Mail: info@hidrex.de

Liposuction aspiration hidrectomy

Dr. Popp, licca Klinik
Hofackerstr. 19, D-86179 Augsburg/Haunstetten
Tel.: +49 (0)8 21/81 55 122, Fax: +49 (0)8 21/81 55 117
http://www.licca.de / E-Mail: popp@licca.de

Medical centers and clinics

Prof. Dr. Dr. Dirk Nolte

Praxisklinik für Mund-, Kiefer- und Gesichtschirurgie
Sauerbruchstr. 48, D-81377 München
Tel.: +49 (0)89/74 80 99 99, Fax: +49 (0)89/74 00 91 35
http:// www.mkg-praxisklinik.com
E-Mail: dirk.nolte@mkg-praxisklinik.com, dirk.nolte@rub.de

Prof. Dr. W. J. Stelter

Städtische Kliniken Frankfurt Hoechst
Gothenstr. 6–8, D-65929 Frankfurt
Tel.: +49 (0)69/31 06 23 23, Fax: +49 (0)69/31 06 24 99
http://skfh.de, E-Mail: chirurgie@skfh.de

PD Dr. Christoph Schick

Deutsches Hyperhidrosezentrum DHHZ (German Hyperhidrosiscenter)
Prinz-Ludwig-Str. 6, D-80333 München
Tel.: +49 (0)89/27 27 20-12, Fax: +49 (0)89/27 27 20-13
http://www.hyperhidrosis.de, E-Mail: schick@hyperhidrosis.de

Prof. Dr. Roland Scola

Wilhelmsburger Krankenhaus „Groß-Sand"
Groß-Sand 3, D-21107 Hamburg
Tel.: +49 (0)40/75 20 53 71, Fax: +49 (0)40/75 20 53 56
http://www.krankenhaus-gross-sand.de
E-Mail: prof.scola@krankenhaus-gross-sand.de

Prof. Dr. Dr. Th. Ruzicka

Universitätshautklinik Düsseldorf
Moorenstr. 5, D-40225 Düsseldorf
Tel.: +49 (0)2 11/811 76 08 (Klinikbüro)
http://www.med.uni-duesseldorf.de
E-Mail: Ruzicka@med.uni-duesseldorf.de
Schweiß-Sprechstunde (nach Vereinbarung)

Prof. Dr. Erhard Hölzle

Klinik für Dermatologie und Allergologie
Klinikum Oldenburg
Dr.-Eden-Str. 10, D-26133 Oldenburg
Tel.: +49 (0)4 41/403 28-50/51, Fax: +49 (0)4 41/403 28-52
http://www.kliniken-oldenburg.de
E-Mail: hoelzle.erhard@kliniken-oldenburg.de

Prof. Dr. med. Marc Heckmann
Praxisklinik für Dermatologie
Kreuzstr. 24, D-82319 Starnberg
Tel.: +49 (0)81 51/95 97-0, Fax: +49 (0)81 51/95 97-22
http://www.derma.de, E-Mail: heckmann@derma.de

Dr. Ivo Tarfusser
Freiheitsstr. 63, I-39012 Meran (BZ)
Tel.: +39 (0)3 35/24 16 86, Fax: +39 (0)4 73/23 64 09
E-Mail: summit@em.parsec.it

PD Dr. Timo Telaranta
St. Anna Klinik
Cavourstr. 58, I-39012 Meran
Tel.: +39 (0)3 33/860 48 15 (personal Hotline)
Fax: +39 (0)4 73/25 63 30
E-Mail: timtel@privatix.fi

PD Dr. med. R. Andresen, Dr. med. Jens Nickel
Abteilung für Bildgebende Diagnostik und Interventionelle Radiologie,
KMG Klinikum Güstrow
Friedrich-Trendelenburg-Allee 1, D-18273 Güstrow
Tel.: +49 (0)38 43/34 27 51, Fax: +49 (0)38 43/343 28 27 51
http://www.kmg.ag, E-Mail: randresen@kmg.ag, jnickel@kmg.ag

Prof. Dr. med. Dr. h.c. mult. Gerd Plewig
Klinik und Poliklinik für Dermatologie und Allergologie
Klinikum der Universität München
Frauenlobstr. 9–11, D-80337 München
Tel.: +49 (0)51 60/61 41, Fax: +49 (0)51 60/61 42
http://www.med.uni-muenchen.de
E-Mail: michael.galinski@med.uni-muenchen.de

Klinik für Dermatologie, Allergologie und Venerologie
Charité Universitätsmedizin Berlin Campus Charité Mitte
Schumannstr. 20–21, D-10117 Berlin (Mitte)
Tel.: +49 (0)30/84 45-69 05, Fax: +49 (0)30/84 45-69 07

Campus Charité Benjamin Franklin
Fabeckstr. 60–62, D-14195 Berlin (Dahlem)
Spezialsprechstunde für übermäßige Schweißproduktion
Tel.: +49 (0)30/84 45-69 05, Fax: +49 (0)30/84 45-69 07

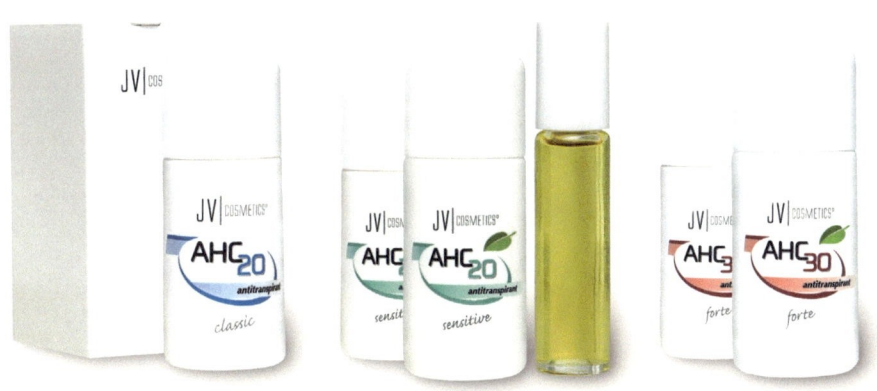

AHC-PRODUCTS

A C Products create a natural seal of the sweat gland orifices in the intermediate and lower layers of skin. The effect appears after the first applications and reduces the secretion of perspiration by 80 to 100%. The sense of well being is not impaired by the treatment since the body still has a sufficient number of evaporation surfaces besides the treated zones. The products, which are exclusively for external use, are highly protective of the skin because of their enrichment with plant extracts. In most cases one application per week is enough.

The company, JV Cosmetics of Switzerland, was established in 1998 with the goal of producing products to counteract excessive perspiration using high-quality ingredients. The striving for higher product efficiency and an acute awareness of costs are parts of the company's philosophy: to be able to offer our customers an optimal ratio of price to performance. JV Cosmetics achieves this by a modern, ISO 9001:2000-certifiierd Process management system; by which all processes [assuring] the optimal development and production of the products desired by our customers are regulated.

Further information: WWW.SCHWITZEN-INFO.CH